Just What the Doctor Ordered

DIABETES COOKBOOK

A Doctor's Approach to Eating Well with Diabetes

JOSEPH D'AMORE, MD, & LISA D'AMORE-MILLER

American Diabetes Association®

Director, Book Publishing, Robert Anthony; *Managing Editor,* Abe Ogden; *Acquisitions Editor,* Victor Van Beuren; *Editor,* Greg Guthrie; *Production Manager,* Melissa Sprott; *Composition,* ADA; *Cover Design,* Vis-à-Vis Creative Concepts, Inc.; *Photographer,* Taran Z.

Printed in Canada
1 3 5 7 9 10 8 6 4 2

The suggestions and information contained in this publication are generally consistent with the *Clinical Practice Recommendations* and other policies of the American Diabetes Association, but they do not represent the policy or position of the Association or any of its boards or committees. Reasonable steps have been taken to ensure the accuracy of the information presented. However, the American Diabetes Association cannot ensure the safety or efficacy of any product or service described in this publication. Individuals are advised to consult a physician or other appropriate health care professional before undertaking any diet or exercise program or taking any medication referred to in this publication. Professionals must use and apply their own professional judgment, experience, and training and should not rely solely on the information contained in this publication before prescribing any diet, exercise, or medication. The American Diabetes Association—its officers, directors, employees, volunteers, and members—assumes no responsibility or liability for personal or other injury, loss, or damage that may result from the suggestions or information in this publication.

♾ The paper in this publication meets the requirements of the ANSI Standard Z39.48-1992 (permanence of paper).

ADA titles may be purchased for business or promotional use or for special sales. To purchase more than 50 copies of this book at a discount, or for custom editions of this book with your logo, contact the American Diabetes Association at the address below, at booksales@diabetes.org, or by calling 703-299-2046.

American Diabetes Association
1701 North Beauregard Street
Alexandria, Virginia 22311

DOI: 10.2337/9781580403351

Library of Congress Cataloging-in-Publication Data

D'Amore, Joseph.
   Just what the doctor ordered diabetes cookbook : a doctor's approach to eating well with diabetes / by Joseph D'Amore & Lisa D'Amore-Miller.
        p. cm.
Includes bibliographical references and index.
ISBN 978-1-58040-335-1 (alk. paper)
1. Diabetes--Diet therapy--Recipes. I. D'Amore-Miller, Lisa. II. Title.
 RC662.D333 2010
 641.5'6314--dc22

                         2010008031

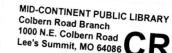
This book is dedicated to my mom,
who taught and encouraged me at a very young age
to play with ingredients and have fun with food.
With her patience and inspiration, she gave me the tools
I needed to be creative and passionate about food
and to enjoy it with family, neighbors, and friends.

I also would like to dedicate a warm thank you to my husband, Ray,
and our children, Stephanie and Christopher. They endured extra
responsibilities as I wore many hats as a full-time wife and mother,
full-time student, and author. I couldn't have done it without their help.

Lisa D'Amore-Miller

Contents

Dr. Joseph D'Amore

I was raised in Brooklyn in the '50s and '60s in a close-knit family whose entire existence revolved around the kitchen. My earliest memories are those of my Hungarian-Jewish grandmother and my Neapolitan grandmother competing in an alliance to fatten up their grandchildren. As the oldest of my brothers and sister and one interested in the entire cooking process, I was often the willing volunteer in many culinary events.

Each grandmother, my mother, and all my aunts took advantage of the easy access to the fresh produce, meats, poultry, and fish available in the region. They used traditional recipes from Eastern Europe and the Italian Mediterranean. Every weekend, holiday, or special occasion was a gourmet festival. Our tables groaned under the weight of herring, chopped liver, fresh pastas, fish, homemade biscotti, stuffed cabbage, antipasto, matzo ball soup, veal and sausage stews, chicken and garlic dishes, and other family favorites.

Every Sunday and for every occasion we ate as a family. Our neighbors would "accidentally" drop by on all of the Italian-American-Jewish holidays, just to sample the food they knew would be on the stove. When 40 people were expected for dinner, it meant we cooked for 80, just to be sure that no one would waste away in the next day or following week.

As I grew up, I became a true foodie and continued to have all the holidays at my house. My wonderful wife, three great kids, nieces, nephews, extended family, and friends can still enjoy the culinary tradition that my Italian and Hungarian grandmothers started 90 years ago. Everyone at my table is family.

Lisa D'Amore-Miller

Growing up on Long Island, I can remember that my mom had full control of the kitchen and that I was her sous chef–mother's little helper. Our entire family gathered every Sunday to eat a five-course meal that lasted all afternoon. Everyone sat around the table, laughing and talking, surrounded by food! My mother encouraged me at a very young age to creatively engage with food. She taught me about recipe development, budgeting, and purchasing. She also taught me how to shop and cook a meal for a large group of people–also known as my family. Her professional training came in the form of feeding a large family. I decided to take my passion for cooking a step further and went to culinary school. It is no big wonder that I graduated at the top of my class, which I credit to Mom and my big brother, Joe, and I continued my education, obtaining a bachelor of science in nutrition. I have the great opportunity to pass down traditional family recipes to my children and create lasting memories with them, as my mother has done with me.

As an established doctor and all-around great cook, Joe is a professional, but most importantly, he is my big brother, who encourages and inspires me to be a better foodie. We are a brother-and-sister team who love to cook fast, simple-to-prepare, healthy meals. As a medical doctor/chef teamed up with a great nutritionist/chef, together we have the experience that qualifies us to provide the educational tools you need to successfully accomplish your goals.

We have a strong family history of diabetes and, although we are currently free of this devastating disorder, we know too well the effects of this growing epidemic. As health care professionals with culinary backgrounds, we offer a combined approach: healthy meals and regular exercise to improve your quality of life.

DIABETES AND YOU

A person with diabetes is unable to secrete adequate insulin, use insulin effectively, or both. Diabetes results either from failure of the pancreas to produce insulin (as in type 1 diabetes) or from insulin resistance, with inadequate insulin secretion to sustain normal metabolism (as in type 2 diabetes). The American Diabetes Association estimates that more than 5 million Americans have diabetes, but don't know it.

About 5–10% of people with diabetes have type 1 diabetes. Although type 1 diabetes can develop at any age, most people are diagnosed when they are under 30 years of age. There is an insulin deficiency in which little if any insulin is secreted, and people with type 1 diabetes will have to take insulin.

The remaining 90–95% of people with diabetes have type 2 diabetes, which used to occur mostly in people aged 40 years or older. However, the rate of type 2 diabetes is increasing in children and adolescents. This disturbing trend is often connected with being overweight or obese, in 80–90% of cases, and with having a family history of diabetes. People with diabetes can still produce their own insulin to varying degrees (some even still produce normal amounts of insulin), but they have become resistant to the effects of insulin. In many cases treatment will require changing diet, changing medications, and increasing physical activity.

Both types of diabetes are treated with meal plans, regular exercise, and medications. Changing food intakes and physical activity patterns are important components that can positively change anyone's physical health, especially for those with diabetes.

Metabolic Syndrome and Pre-Diabetes

The metabolic syndrome is a cluster of metabolic disorders that is characterized by obesity and insulin resistance. Other components of the metabolic syndrome include high cholesterol, high blood pressure, and abnormal blood glucose levels. People who have the metabolic syndrome are at greater risk for developing cardiovascular disease and type 2 diabetes in the future.

When a person's blood glucose levels are abnormal, but not high enough to clinically diagnose diabetes, then that person is considered to have pre-diabetes, sometimes referred to as impaired fasting glucose or impaired glucose tolerance (this is also a factor of the metabolic syndrome). When someone has pre-diabetes, he or she is at greater risk of developing diabetes. It is important to have a doctor check for pre-diabetes. Having pre-diabetes means the pancreas has already started to show signs of strain. Even when blood glucose is just slightly elevated, the condition can begin damaging the heart and circulatory system.

To fully understand the metabolic syndrome, pre-diabetes, and diabetes, it is important to understand insulin resistance. When we eat, sugar is released into the bloodstream, making our blood glucose levels rise. The job of the hormone insulin, which is produced by beta cells in the pancreas, is to move the glucose from the blood into the body's cells to be used for energy. But when we have insulin resistance, the cells in our body are impaired and are less efficient at using insulin. This means the body has less energy available to function properly. The pancreas secretes enough additional insulin to overcome the resistance for a while; however, the pancreas can become "exhausted" over time, and eventually supply cannot keep up with demand. This is when blood glucose levels become elevated.

NUTRITION AND DIABETES

Planning a Healthy Diet

Following a healthy, balanced meal plan is everyone's goal because it can help get blood glucose levels under control. A healthy, balanced meal plan involves planning a menu and purchasing and preparing seasonal foods. The goal in meal planning is to meet the body's nutritional requirements, not just satisfy what tickles your taste buds.

Don't confuse healthy eating with dieting. The word "diet" may make you cringe because many people associate it with eating less or not eating what they like, but healthy eating with diabetes is focused on eating well, not eating with restrictions. Healthy eating is a lifestyle, not a temporary "diet." It involves making wise food choices, incorporating variety in what you eat, eating in moderation, and making small changes in how you eat.

An apple a day may not necessarily keep the doctor away if an apple is the only fruit you eat. Remember, variety is one of the keys to healthy eating. By eating a variety of foods, you will be able to add new, exciting flavors to your meals, and you will benefit from a diversity of nutrients. So switch it up, and try something new!

There are no "bad" or "forbidden" foods in a healthy meal plan. The key is moderation. You can have your cake and eat it too, so long as you make space in your meal plan for that slice of cake and don't go overboard at dessert. One of the keys to building a healthy meal plan is to coordinate what you are eating with a registered dietitian, especially one who has expertise in diabetes. He or she will let you know exactly how many carbohydrates, calories, and fat grams you should be eating every day. Once you know that information, you can start to make space in your meal plan for the foods you love, although sometimes you'll have to choose healthier versions of those favorites. For example, you may have to choose smaller portions of baked potato chips instead of your old favorite fat-laden chips.

The road to a healthy meal plan involves some easy changes. Choose 100% whole-wheat bread over white bread. Eat a piece of fruit instead of drinking fruit juice. Start reading food labels on the foods you buy. Watch *how much* you eat, not just *what* you eat. Simple changes like these can help with blood glucose levels and help you lose weight.

Here's a huge tool in changing eating into healthy eating: eat at home more often. That's where cookbooks like *Just What the Doctor Ordered* can help you. Try preparing a new recipe every day. Many people wrongly believe that healthy eating is an "all or nothing" prospect: unless you completely stop eating all of the foods you love, you will not achieve your weight-loss goals. As you will see from the recipes in this book, that is far from the truth. By shopping for healthy ingredients, preparing wholesome meals at home, and eating reasonable portions with your loved ones, you can make a healthy meal plan not only a part of your life, but also a part that you enjoy!

Plate Presentation:
A Prescription for Success

Throughout this book, you will see recipes with a Prescription for Success. Keep an eye out for these helpful hints. An important and often overlooked aspect of menu planning is presentation. People are more likely to eat and enjoy foods that appeal to the senses in some way or another. This goes beyond just taste. Presentation covers the colors, shapes, textures, temperature, and smells of a dish. Use these Prescriptions for Success to thrill your senses, so you will want to enjoy these healthy recipes again and again.

Color can help create eye-catching dishes. Colorful fruits and vegetables can help you create a pleasing appearance on your plates. For example, if you have a dish with a white crème sauce, use orange segments to offer a contrasting color and make the meal more inviting to the eye. Using color in your main dishes or as garnish is a vital part of menu planning.

Using shapes can also please the senses of your diners. There are so many options. You can slice zucchini *julienne*, which is a 2-inch thin cut, or slice a potato *allumette*, which is also a 2-inch cut but thicker. These different shapes draw the eye and make people want to taste these pretty, creative dishes—including you. There are other ways to get innovative shapes into your dishes: grating, peeling, curling, twisting, and dicing.

Contrasting sizes and shapes are important to creating an appealing dish. When making a dish that

(continued on p. 4)

(continued from p. 3)

contains several similar ingredients, it is best to cut all of the pieces the same size. If the plate serves a chunky cut of meat, for example, it may be best to offer long, lean asparagus or allumette-cut vegetables. Plated food that shows height also adds visual interest. If you're looking to be innovative in your presentation, try building up instead of out to the ends of the plate. To help keep food interesting, be creative and offer different ways to present each of your food dishes.

Texture adds excitement to any meal. Combining crispness with soft, smooth textures is nearly always a successful outcome. Crispy toasted pita bread served with a smooth vegetable bean dip is a pleasurable combination. When granola is added to yogurt, the combination of textures makes the dish feel like a complete meal.

Temperature adds interest and drama to a meal. Think of a cold, crisp tossed salad with warm, grilled chicken breast or a hot roll with cool jam or jelly. Sounds delightful, right? Some foods are naturally hot, like a jalapeño pepper, or cool, like peppermint. Seasonings that offer a temperature difference are a great resource for creative cooking.

Flavor characteristics include sweet, salty, sour, and bitter. These characteristics are recognized at different areas of the tongue. But it is with our noses, however, that we first sense "flavor." Meals are more interesting when we incorporate both delicate and robust flavors. A bland meal is boring; variety is important to draw the attention of the tongue and the nose.

Healthy Behaviors and Habits

One of the hardest, but most important, tactics for eating healthier meals is to change your habits and behaviors, particularly those that surround food and eating. Eating too many high-fat and high-calorie foods and not getting enough exercise are associated with unhealthy lifestyle choices. Often, lifestyle habits come from our cultures and traditions and personal desires, but these behaviors can be changed if you are enthusiastic, interested, and committed. People do not lose weight and keep it off if they follow a healthy meal plan for just one month; they must make healthy eating a part of how they live.

To make positive changes in your lifestyle, you'll need to focus on physical activity and a healthful meal plan, not magic potions and fad diets.

Variety Is the Spice of Life

A balanced diet requires that you consume enough of each type of food without overdoing it. Following a balanced diet gets you nearly all of the essential nutrients that you need to stay healthy. Even more, a balanced diet gets you variety in what you eat. Variety is the spice of life! You may enjoy peaches today, apples in Waldorf salad tomorrow, and a fruit parfait the day after that. Maybe you want a breakfast burrito today, navy beans in vegetable pesto soup tomorrow, and the three-bean salad the day after that. Eating a variety of foods will keep your taste buds happy.

You've no doubt heard about balanced diets ever since you were a child and used the old food pyramid to help you build a healthy diet. Recently, the U.S. Food and Drug Administration revised its old food pyramid and created a new system called MyPyramid that allows you to know precisely how many servings of each food group you should be eating per day. This new system is personalized for your needs across activity levels, age, and eating habits. You can see the MyPyramid at www.mypyramid.gov.

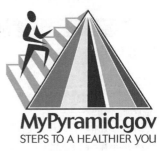

Shop Smart

Smart shopping can save you money and net you valuable, healthy nutrients. Have you ever noticed the layout of a supermarket? All the fresh produce, meat, fish, and dairy are located along the perimeter of the store. Canned, boxed, and prepackaged foods are down the aisles. Go shopping with a grocery list that you've put together from your meal plan, and never shop on an empty stomach. So the next time you're in the grocery store, shop around the perimeter of the market first and only hit the aisles later with your list in hand.

Food Choices

Not all eating decisions have to be difficult. Sometimes, the easiest way to better health involves a quick comparison and an equally quick choice. Rather than making a poor food choice, think about what you're about to eat or drink for a moment and make the healthier choice. The following table shows just a few examples of everyday foods compared with better options. Just so you know that you've made the right decision, the benefit column shows why you'll be better off by making the healthy choice.

FOOD	BETTER CHOICE	BENEFIT
8 oz cola	8 oz diet cola	Less carbohydrate Fewer calories
Whole milk	Fat-free milk	Less saturated fat Fewer calories Less cholesterol
Juice	Whole fruit	More fiber
Cheeseburger with French fries	Hamburger with plain baked potato	Less saturated fat and *trans* fat Less cholesterol Less sodium More fiber
Fried chicken with skin on	Skinless roasted chicken	Less saturated fat and *trans* fat Fewer calories Less cholesterol

FOOD	BETTER CHOICE	BENEFIT
Mayonnaise	Fat-free mayonnaise	Fewer calories Less fat Less saturated fat Less cholesterol
Potato salad	Three-bean salad	More fiber
White bread	100% whole-wheat bread	More fiber
Pizza with pepperoni	Pizza with vegetables	More nutrients Less saturated fat Fewer calories Less sodium
Potato chips	Pretzels	Less fat
Ice cream	Frozen yogurt	Less saturated fat Fewer calories

Portion Control

It's not just all about what you eat. A healthy meal plan also focuses on how much you eat. Even if you're eating the healthiest food on the planet, if you eat too much of it, you will gain weight. The best way to figure out how much you're eating is to actually measure your food. So when you're cooking at home, break out those measuring cups and measuring spoons, so you know precisely how much you're eating. Plus, when your measurements are exact, you'll be cooking better dishes, because the flavors will be in the right proportions. It also doesn't hurt to get a kitchen scale for your foods, so you can know exactly how much chicken, pasta, or flour you're using in a recipe.

If you're not eating at home and you don't want to carry along all of your measuring tools, then you'll have to visualize your portion sizes. Comparing portion sizes with common objects is a helpful alternative to guesstimating what's on your plate.

- Thumb = 1 oz cheese
- Marshmallow = 2 Tbsp peanut butter
- Golf ball = 2 Tbsp salad dressing; 1/4 cup dried fruit
- Deck of cards = 3 oz meat
- Palm of hand = 3 oz
- An ice cream scoop = 1/2 cup
- Baseball = 1 cup fruit or vegetables; 1 cup ready-to-eat cereal; large apple or orange

Defuse Food Cravings

People eat for a variety of reasons, but not always because of hunger. The desire to eat can be triggered by signals other than hunger, even when the body does not need food. These food cravings can occur when we feel bored, anxious, or stressed. Some people have food cravings in response to external cues, such as the time of day, the sight or the smell of a food, or simply from sitting in front of the television. Here are some ways to defuse those food cravings.

KEEP A FOOD DIARY: Recording everything you eat, including the portion sizes, helps you keep track of your calorie and nutrient intakes. Paying attention to what you eat can tip you off to behaviors that lead to weight gain and unexplained blood glucose levels.

PLAN FOR THE OCCASIONAL SLICE OF PIE: Depriving yourself can actually trigger overeating. Making any foods off-limits just increases its allure. Don't completely cut out the food that you love; instead, remember to limit how much of it you eat. Moderation is the key to success.

AMAZING GRAZING: Although eating regularly helps prevent feeling deprived and hungry, grazing can easily add unwanted calories to your meal plan. You know what grazing is: it's when you intend to eat only a few pieces of a food, such as candy, but instead go back again and again, until you've eaten far more than you ever intended. Plan to eat four to six small meals each day, and avoid going long stretches without eating, which can trigger an eating binge.

EAT FOR REAL: Eat all of your meals at the dining table. If you eat while standing up or while sitting in front of the television or computer, you are not paying attention to how much or how quickly you're eating. Eat slowly, put your fork down between bites, and be mindful of satiation. Take this time to reconnect with your family.

EXPECT THE UNEXPECTED: Tempting foods are more likely to trigger over-eating when we come across them unexpectedly. Have healthy snacks on hand to protect yourself from unwanted surprises.

IDENTIFY THE STRESS: If stress makes you overeat, identify what leads to that stress. Respond to the actual problem rather than resorting to food. You may need the help of a registered dietitian or mental health profes-sional to address these powerful urges.

GROUP EFFORT: Group support programs, such as Weight Watchers or group nutrition counseling, can be very helpful in teaching you how to tackle food cravings.

Reading Food Labels

If you're going to be following a healthy meal plan, you first need to know what you're eating. The easiest way to do that is to start reading food labels. They're on nearly everything you buy at the grocery store, so it's time to start paying attention to this vital information and use this ubiquitous tool. Your health will thank you for it.

The U.S. Food and Drug Administration has required that nearly all foods contain a Nutrition Facts label since 1995. You'll find invaluable nutrition information on this little label that will make meal planning a breeze. Although you could spend a long time scrutinizing every detail on a label, it's best to keep an eye out for a few key items: serving size and number of servings, calories, total fat, total carbohydrate, sodium, fiber, and ingredients.

Nutrition Facts

Serving Size 3/4 cup (28g)
Servings Per Container 14

Amount Per Serving

Calories 110   Calories from Fat 9

                % Daily Value*

Total Fat 1g	**2%**
Saturated Fat 0g	**0%**
Trans Fat 0g	
Cholesterol 0mg	**0%**
Sodium 250mg	**10%**
Total Carbohydrate 30g	**10%**
Dietary Fiber 2g	**9%**
Sugars 28g	
Protein 2g	

Vitamin A 0%	•	Vitamin C 25%
Calcium 2%	•	Iron 6%

*Percent Daily Values are based on a 2,000 calorie diet. Your Daily Values may be higher or lower depending on your calorie needs.

	Calories:	2,000	2,500
Total Fat	Less than	65g	80g
Sat Fat	Less than	20g	25g
Cholesterol	Less than	300mg	300mg
Sodium	Less than	2,400mg	2,400mg
Total Carbohydrate		300g	375g
Dietary Fiber		25g	30g

Calories per gram:
Fat 9 • Carbohydrate 4 • Protein 4

INGREDIENTS: WHOLE GRAIN ROLLED OATS, SUGAR, CANOLA OIL, SALT, BAKING SODA, NATURAL FLAVOR, SULFUR DIOXIDE ADDED AS A PRESERVATIVE.

Serving Size and Number of Servings

For people who are trying to lower their intake of carbohydrate, calories, and/or fat intake, this is the very first place to look. All of the information contained in the food label applies to *one serving only*. Therefore, you need to know how many servings there are in a package of food. If there are multiple servings in a package of food, then you will get the amount of nutrients described in the food label for every serving you eat. In the food label on p. 8, the number of calories per serving is 110, but there are 14 servings in the container. If you were to eat that entire container, then you'd be taking in a whopping 1,540 calories!

Thankfully, the food label makes things easier for you. Rather than looking at a package and guessing how you're going to get 14 servings out of it, the label tells you what you need to know. For the food label on p. 8, the serving size is 3/4 cup. If you keep your serving sizes at 3/4 cup, then you will match the nutrients described in the rest of the label for that serving. You'll also get 14 servings out of the container, which can help save you some money!

Calories

If you are trying to lose weight, then you'll need to keep track of how many calories you eat. To lose weight, you need to eat fewer calories than your body burns. Use the food label to know exactly how many calories you're getting with a serving of food and to compare products to choose the one with fewer calories. To find out how many calories you need each day, talk with your dietitian or certified diabetes educator.

Serving Size versus Exchange List Serving Size

Some people use Exchanges/ Choices to help plan their diabetes meal plan. This innovative method of meal planning organizes similar foods into categories or lists. Every food in each list is nutritionally similar and can therefore be exchanged for other foods in that list. Because the foods are organized by nutritional content rather than size of the serving, individual foods on the exchange lists will have different serving sizes. In the vegetables list, for example, a vegetable exchange consists of 25 calories and 5 grams of carbohydrate, which you can receive from either 1/2 cup cooked vegetables or 1 cup salad greens.

If you use this system to help plan your meals, then it's important to recognize that the serving size on a food label is not necessarily the same as an exchange list serving size. Check the labels, and compare them to the exchange information. You many need to adjust your serving size to meet your meal plan needs.

If you're interested in using this method for planning your meals, contact a registered dietitian or purchase a copy of *Choose Your Foods: Exchange Lists for Diabetes* at http://store.diabetes.org.

Total Fat

Total fat tells you how much fat is in a food per serving. It includes the healthier mono- and polyunsaturated fats as well as the less healthy saturated and *trans* fats. Unsaturated fats tend to come from nuts and certain oils (such as canola, olive, and safflower oil), and they can help lower cholesterol and protect the heart. Saturated and *trans* fats can raise cholesterol levels and increase the risk of heart disease. These unhealthy fats are unfortunately all over the place. They are found in butter, lard, ice cream, ground beef, bacon, and cream sauces, to name a few.

Fat is packed with calories, too. Per gram of fat eaten, you'll get 9 calories. So if you're trying to lose weight, cutting out the fat is a great place to start.

Total Carbohydrate

Foods that contain carbohydrate raise blood glucose. By keeping track of how many carbohydrates you eat and setting a limit for your maximum amount to eat, you can help keep your blood glucose levels in your target range. On the label, Total Carbohydrate includes starches, sugars, and fiber.

If you are carbohydrate counting, look at the grams of total carbohydrate, rather than the grams of sugar. If you look only at the amount of sugar, you may end up passing over nutritious foods such as fruits and milks because they appear to be too high in sugar. You might also overeat certain foods, such as cereals and grains that have no natural or added sugar, but do contain a lot of carbohydrate.

Fiber

Fiber is the structural part of plants, found in grains, fruits, and vegetables. Your body cannot digest fiber, so when you consume dietary fiber, most of it just passes through the intestines and leaves the body. As fiber passes through the body, it absorbs water and swells, making you feel full and satiated, which helps you eat less food. It also helps with digestion by cleaning out the system and removing bulk. Because fiber comes from plants, you can't get it from animal products, such as milk, eggs, meat, poultry, and fish.

For good health, adults should try to eat 25–30 grams of fiber every day. Most Americans do not get anywhere close to enough fiber in their diets, so any increase in fiber intake can be beneficial. Increasing your intake of fiber can help prevent heart disease because it lowers cholesterol levels. Most of us only get about half of what is recommended. Fiber can be found in whole grains, fruits, vegetables, and legumes.

Sodium

Sodium does not affect blood glucose levels. However, many people consume far more sodium than they need. Table salt, for example, is very high in sodium. With many foods, you can taste how salty they are, such as pickles or bacon. But there is also hidden salt in many foods, such as cheeses, salad dressings, canned soups, and other packaged foods. Use food labels to compare the sodium in different foods. Try using herbs and spices rather than adding salt. Adults should aim for less than 2,300 mg of sodium per day. If you have high blood pressure, you may want to consume even less sodium.

Ingredients

Ingredients are listed in descending order by weight, meaning the first ingredient makes up the largest proportion of the food. Check the ingredient list to spot things you want to avoid, such as coconut oil or palm oil, which are high in saturated fat. Also try to avoid hydrogenated oils that are high in *trans* fat.

The ingredient list is also a good place to look for heart-healthy ingredients such as soy; monounsaturated fats such as olive, canola, or peanut oils; or whole grains, such as whole-wheat flour and oats.

Nutrient Claims

Nutrient claims may be used on labels as long as they meet the U.S. Food and Drug Administration definitions. Nutrient claims such as "cholesterol free" and "low in fat" include the conditions under which each term can be used. For example, a cholesterol-free product may have less than 2 milligrams of cholesterol and may not contain more than 2 grams of saturated fat and *trans* fat combined per serving.

Reliable food label health claims include "diets low in sodium may reduce the risk of high blood pressure" and "diets high in fruits and vegetables may reduce the risk of cancer." The FDA examines scientific evidence from food manufacturers and establishes a clear link between diet and health.

Unlike health claims, structure-function claims can be made without FDA approval as long as there is no mention of a disease or symptom. Examples of structure-function claims include "supports heart health," "builds strong bones," and "slows aging." These are not as reliable.

Sugar Substitutes

Many people turn to alternative sweeteners to help control calories and limit sugar intake. There are four artificial sweeteners approved by the FDA, including saccharin, acesulfame-K, sucralose, and aspartame. Stevia is an herbal alternative to artificial sweeteners and was granted FDA approval in 2008.

There are also sugar replacers, which are sometimes referred to as nutritive sweeteners. Sugar replacers are also called sugar alcohols. Some examples include xylitol, mannitol, sorbitol, and lactitol. Sugar alcohols contain fewer calories and less carbohydrate than the other sweeteners. Many of these are used in foods labeled as "no sugar added," such as ice creams, cookies, puddings, and candy. The body absorbs sugar alcohols slowly. Side effects such as gas, abdominal discomfort, and diarrhea make them less attractive to consumers than artificial sweeteners. Another problem with some of these sweeteners is that people get used to the high sweetness factor and find it difficult to use regular sugar in moderation.

Sweetener Name	Brand Names	Sweetness Factor
SACCHARIN	Sweet'N Low, Sweet Twin, Sugar Twin	300×
ACESULFAME-K	Sunett, Sweet One	180–200×
SUCRALOSE	Splenda	600×
ASPARTAME	NutraSweet, Equal	180×
STEVIA	PureVia, Truvia, SweetLeaf	300×
ERYTHRITOL	Zsweet, Sun Crystals	70% as sweet as sugar
XYLITOL	XyloSweet	Same as sugar

PHYSICAL ACTIVITY

Physical activity is an important part of treating diabetes. Exercise can make the body use insulin more effectively. It makes the heart stronger, improves circulation, and lowers blood pressure. It raises the level of HDL or "good" cholesterol in your blood. It improves muscle tone and strength. Exercise can relieve stress, depression, and tension; improve your mood; and improve how much and how well you sleep. Exercise can improve self-confidence and boost self-esteem.

For people with type 1 diabetes, exercise is always balanced with a meal plan and insulin to manage blood glucose levels. Changes may have to be made in insulin or food intake or both before and after exercise to prevent low blood glucose levels.

For people with type 2 diabetes, exercise helps increase the body cells' sensitivity to insulin. With this increased sensitivity, insulin works better and blood glucose levels improve. The more often a person exercises, the more likely it is that this will happen. In many people with type 2 diabetes, exercise is combined with a meal plan and possibly medications to manage the diabetes.

Choose an exercise routine that will fit with your lifestyle and physical abilities. Experts recommend that people set a goal of exercising at moderate intensity for 30–60 minutes for 5–7 days per week. However, it can be broken into only three to four 15-minute exercise sessions per day. Try to make exercise a part of your daily life. It is better to walk 30 minutes every day than 2 hours once a week!

Many people with diabetes get great benefits from aerobic exercise. Sustained aerobic exercise can use large amounts of energy. Examples of aerobic exercise are walking, running, bicycling, and swimming. These methods of exercise are more likely to help you manage your blood glucose than activities that require only short bursts of energy, like many team sports and some calisthenics. While you're at it, don't forget the value of strength training and stretching. Strength training, such as lifting weights, will build muscle, which helps your body more effectively manage blood glucose levels. Stretching is helpful in that it increases flexibility and reduces the risk of exercise-related injuries.

Exercise Tips

- **See your doctor.** You should consult with your doctor before beginning an exercise routine.
- **Test yourself.** Your doctor will tell you when to test your blood glucose when you exercise, depending on how you exercise and for how long.
- **Take insulin if you need it.** If you are on insulin, your doctor might change your insulin dosage for exercise or sports.
- **Eat right.** Your doctor will also help you figure out what to eat to keep going. You might need extra snacks before, during, or after exercise.
- **Bring snacks and liquids.** Whether you're playing a football game at school or swimming in your backyard, you should have snacks and water nearby.
- **Pack it up.** If you will be exercising away from home, pack testing supplies, medications, your medical alert bracelet, emergency contact information, and a copy of your diabetes management plan.
- **Tell your coaches.** If you're playing organized sports, be sure that your coaches know about your diabetes. Tell them the things that you need to do to control diabetes before, during, or after a game.

- **Take control.** You're in control of your health. Stop playing a sport or exercising if you need to drink water, eat a snack for low blood glucose, go to the bathroom, or check your glucose levels. Also, stop if you feel any signs that something is wrong.
- **Be safe.** Do not exercise if your blood glucose is over 200 mg/dl, your fasting glucose is over 180 mg/dl, or if you have ketones in your urine.

Blood Glucose Levels and Exercise

During exercise, your body uses more glucose for energy than when your body is at rest. This can result in a rapid lowering of your blood glucose if you are taking insulin or an oral diabetes medicine that lowers blood glucose levels. It is important that you keep your blood glucose in a safe range while you exercise. In order to do this, there must be a balance between the glucose used for energy while you exercise, the glucose available from food, and any diabetes medications taken to lower your blood glucose. Testing blood glucose is the best way to check this balance.

Always be prepared for low blood glucose when exercising. Sometimes hypoglycemia is harder to recognize when you are exercising. Test your blood glucose level if you become sweaty or lightheaded or if you experience any other signs of hypoglycemia. If possible, exercise with a family member or friend who can help if necessary. Always carry some form of identification that indicates that you have diabetes. When you exercise, bring along some form of quick-acting carbohydrate, such as glucose tablets, glucose gel, or fruit juice.

If you are starting a new exercise routine, like training for a sport, your doctor might change your insulin or medication dosage to prevent these problems. Also, keep an eye on cuts, scrapes, or blisters, and be sure to tell your doctor right away if they are really red, swollen, or ooze pus–they might be infected, which can be very dangerous.

Symptoms of Hypoglycemia and Hyperglycemia

Hypoglycemia/ low blood glucose

You may have low blood glucose if you are
- Sweating
- Lightheaded
- Shaky
- Weak
- Anxious
- Hungry
- Having a headache
- Having difficulty concentrating
- Confused

Hyperglycemia/ high blood glucose

You may have high blood glucose if you:
- Feel very thirsty
- Have to urinate a lot
- Feel very tired
- Have blurry vision

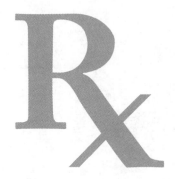

Breakfast

Whole-Wheat Gingerbread Waffles

1/2 cup	all-purpose flour
1/2 cup	whole-wheat flour
1 Tbsp	granulated sugar
1 Tbsp	brown sugar
1/2 tsp	baking powder
1 tsp	ground ginger
1/4 tsp	ground cinnamon

❖ Mix together flours, sugars, baking powder, ginger, and cinnamon in a large bowl.

1 cup	nonfat milk
2 Tbsp	margarine, melted

❖ In a separate bowl, mix milk and margarine until well blended. Gradually add milk mixture to flour mixture, stirring until batter is smooth.

2	large egg whites

❖ Beat egg whites until soft peaks form. Fold egg whites into batter.

	nonstick cooking spray

❖ Preheat and spray waffle iron with cooking spray. Follow the waffle iron's instructions for how much batter to use and how long to cook it, usually between 2 and 4 minutes or until steam stops escaping.

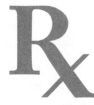

Exchanges/Choices
2 Starch • 1 Fat

Calories 200 • Calories from Fat 40 • Total Fat 4.5g • Saturated Fat 1.1g • Trans Fat 0.0g • Cholesterol 0mg • Sodium 145mg • Total Carbohydrate 33g • Dietary Fiber 2g • Sugars 10g • Protein 8g

Chunky Apple Muffins

Serves 18 / Serving size: 1 muffin

18	paper cupcake liners

❖ Preheat oven to 350°F, and line cupcake pan with paper liners.

1 1/2 cups	granulated sugar
1 Tbsp	vanilla
2	large eggs

❖ Mix sugar, vanilla, and eggs in a large bowl.

1 1/2 cups	all-purpose flour
1 Tbsp	cinnamon
1 tsp	baking soda
1 tsp	baking powder
1/2 tsp	salt

❖ In a separate bowl, combine flour, cinnamon, baking soda, baking powder, and salt.

2 cups	McIntosh apples, peeled and chopped
2 cups	Granny Smith apples, peeled and chopped

❖ Using an electric mixer on low speed, mix dry ingredients into egg mixture. Fold in apples. Fill each muffin cup 3/4 full, and bake 25 minutes.

Prescription for Success

Try these variations:
- Raisin Spice Muffin: fold 10 oz raisins and 1 1/4 tsp allspice to mixture
- Pear Muffins: substitute apples for pears
- Pecan Apple Cake Muffin: fold 3 Tbsp chopped pecans into mixture

Exchanges/Choices

2 Carbohydrate

Calories 125 • Calories from Fat 5 • Total Fat 0.5g • Saturated Fat 0.2g • Trans Fat 0.0g • Cholesterol 25mg • Sodium 165mg • Total Carbohydrate 29g • Dietary Fiber 1g • Sugars 20g • Protein 2g

Bran Muffins

12	paper cupcake liners

❖ Preheat oven to 375°F. Place cupcake liners in pan.

2	large eggs
1 cup	low-fat buttermilk
1/3 cup	packed brown sugar
1/4 cup	canola oil
1/3 cup	molasses

❖ In a large bowl, beat eggs; then add buttermilk, brown sugar, oil, and molasses.

1 1/4 cups	whole-wheat flour
1 cup	natural bran cereal
1 tsp	baking soda
1/2 tsp	baking powder
1/2 tsp	salt
3/4 cup	raisins

❖ In a separate bowl, combine flour, bran, baking soda, baking powder, and salt. Stir flour mixture into egg mixture until smooth. Fold in raisins.

❖ Spoon batter into prepared muffin cups until 3/4 full. Bake for 25 minutes or until tops spring back when lightly touched. Let cool 10 minutes. Remove from pan, and cool on racks.

Prescription for Success

Try these variations

- Apple Bran Muffin: add 1/2 cup chopped apples and 1/2 cup applesauce
- Raisin Bran Muffin: add 1 cup golden raisins
- Chocolate Chip Bran Muffins: add 1 cup chocolate chips

Exchanges/Choices

2 Carbohydrate • 1 Fat

Calories 190 • Calories from Fat 55 • Total Fat 6.0g • Saturated Fat 0.8g • Trans Fat 0.0g • Cholesterol 35mg • Sodium 280mg • Total Carbohydrate 33g • Dietary Fiber 2g • Sugars 18g • Protein 4g

Whole-Wheat Pancakes

1/2 cup	all-purpose flour
1/2 cup	whole-wheat flour
2 Tbsp	brown sugar
2 Tbsp	baking powder

❖ In a medium bowl, stir together flours, brown sugar, and baking powder.

1	egg
3/4 cup	nonfat milk
2 Tbsp	margarine, melted

❖ In a separate bowl, combine egg, milk, and melted margarine. Add flour mixture to egg mixture; batter will be lumpy.

	nonstick cooking spray

❖ Lightly spray griddle or heavy skillet with cooking spray. For each pancake, pour 1/4 cup pancake batter. Cook pancakes until the tops are full of bubbles and begin to look dry, and bottoms are golden brown. Turn and brown the other side.

Prescription for Success
Top each serving with 1/2 cup fresh sliced strawberries and 1 Tbsp pancake syrup.

Exchanges/Choices
2 Starch • 1 Fat

Calories 205 • Calories from Fat 55 • Total Fat 6.0g • Saturated Fat 1.5g • Trans Fat 0.0g • Cholesterol 55mg • Sodium 630mg • Total Carbohydrate 34g • Dietary Fiber 2g • Sugars 9g • Protein 7g

Phyllo Egg and Veggie Packages

Serves 4 / Serving size: 2 packages

| | nonstick cooking spray |

❖ Preheat oven to 350°F.

❖ Spray a cupcake pan with cooking spray.

| 16 | 9 × 14-inch phyllo sheets |

❖ Lightly spray each phyllo sheet with cooking spray. Place two sheets into each cupcake cup to form a cup.

12 oz	egg substitute
4 Tbsp	chopped mushrooms
1	small zucchini, chopped
2 oz	reduced-fat cheddar cheese

❖ Pour in 1 1/2 oz egg substitute for each serving. Top each cup with mushrooms, zucchini, and cheese. Cover with overlapping phyllo. Bake for 10 minutes, until phyllo cups are lightly browned.

Prescription for Success
Serve with sliced orange wedges.

Exchanges/Choices
2 Starch • 2 Lean Meat

Calories 225 • Calories from Fat 20 • Total Fat 2.5g • Saturated Fat 0.8g • Trans Fat 0.0g • Cholesterol 5mg • Sodium 460mg • Total Carbohydrate 33g • Dietary Fiber 1g • Sugars 2g • Protein 17g

Vegetable Omelet Pita

3	whole-wheat pitas, sliced in half lengthwise

❖ Toast pita halves until golden brown.

6	large eggs
1	small green pepper, chopped
1	small onion, minced
6 oz	mushrooms, sliced

❖ In a medium bowl, whisk together eggs, pepper, onion, and mushrooms.

	nonstick cooking spray
12	cherry tomatoes, halved
3 oz	reduced-fat cheddar cheese, grated

❖ Spray a sauté pan with cooking spray, and heat on medium. Pour mixture into sauté pan, cook for 3 minutes. Add tomatoes, turn omelet over, sprinkle with cheese, and cook for 2 minutes longer. Place each pita half on a plate, and top with omelet.

Prescription for Success
For an extra kick, substitute low-fat Monterey Jack cheese for the cheddar.

Exchanges/Choices
1 Starch • 1 Vegetable • 1 Med-Fat Meat • 1/2 Fat

Calories 195 • Calories from Fat 65 • Total Fat 7.0g • Saturated Fat 2.4g • Trans Fat 0.0g • Cholesterol 215mg • Sodium 320mg • Total Carbohydrate 20g • Dietary Fiber 3g • Sugars 3g • Protein 15g

Fruit Crêpe
with Crème Anglaise Sauce

1/2 cup	nonfat milk
1/2 cup	all-purpose flour
1/4 tsp	salt
1	large egg
1 Tbsp	margarine, melted
	nonstick cooking spray

❖ Combine all ingredients in a bowl. Mix thoroughly. Heat a small (5-inch) pan on medium, and lightly coat with cooking spray. Pour 1/4 cup batter in pan, and circulate pan to coat the entire bottom. Cook each crêpe until they begin to look dry and the bottom is light brown. Turn and brown the other side.

1/2 cup	nonfat milk
1 1/2 Tbsp	arrowroot

❖ In a small bowl, mix milk with arrowroot to form a slurry.

1/2 cup	nonfat milk
1/4 cup	granulated sugar
1 tsp	vanilla extract
1 tsp	almond extract

❖ In a saucepan over medium heat, warm milk until small bubbles form. Do not boil. Gradually pour arrowroot slurry into the warm milk, stirring constantly. Add sugar and vanilla and almond extracts. Whisk until mixture is thick enough to coat a spoon.

3/4 lb	peaches, peeled and sliced

❖ Reserve half of the Anglaise sauce on the side, and keep warm. Add the peaches to the remaining sauce. Stir until well coated, about 3 minutes. Spoon the peach mixture into crêpes, and top with reserved sauce.

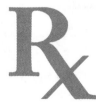

Exchanges/Choices
2 1/2 Carbohydrate • 1/2 Fat

Calories 215 • Calories from Fat 30 • Total Fat 3.5g • Saturated Fat 1.0g • Trans Fat 0.0g • Cholesterol 55mg • Sodium 225mg • Total Carbohydrate 39g • Dietary Fiber 1g • Sugars 24g • Protein 7g

Yogurt Parfait

1/2 cup	sliced strawberries
1/4 cup	blueberries
1/4 cup	blackberries
1/4 cup	raspberries

❖ Wash berries, and pat dry with a paper towel.

3 cups	plain nonfat yogurt
1	medium ripe banana, sliced

❖ Layer ingredients by placing 1/4 cup yogurt in four individual serving glasses. Top with strawberries, then with 1/4 cup yogurt, top with banana slices, and then with remaining yogurt.

4 Tbsp	wheat germ

❖ Sprinkle each with wheat germ. Finally, top with blueberries, blackberries, and raspberries. Serve cold.

Prescription for Success

Berries contain antioxidants, which help your body fight against free radicals.

Exchanges/Choices

1 Fruit • 1 Fat-Free Milk

Calories 165 • Calories from Fat 15 • Total Fat 1.5g • Saturated Fat 0.4g • Trans Fat 0.0g • Cholesterol 5mg • Sodium 120mg • Total Carbohydrate 28g • Dietary Fiber 3g • Sugars 19g • Protein 12g

Eggs, Spinach, and Caramelized Onions with Potatoes

	nonstick cooking spray
2	*large onions, thinly sliced*
3 Tbsp	*balsamic vinegar*
1 Tbsp	*brown sugar*

❖ Preheat a sauté pan, and lightly spray with cooking spray. Add onions, balsamic vinegar, and brown sugar. Stir frequently for 15 minutes.

6 cups	*spinach, rinsed well and patted dry*

❖ Add spinach and cook until wilted, about 5 minutes, stirring frequently.

2 Tbsp	*olive oil*
3 cups	*peeled and cubed potatoes*
2 tsp	*black pepper*

❖ Meanwhile, in a separate sauté pan over medium heat, add oil. When oil is hot, add potatoes, and cook until lightly browned. Season with pepper.

6	*large eggs*

❖ In a large bowl, whisk eggs, and then pour eggs into a preheated sauté pan coated with cooking spray. Cook thoroughly by flipping eggs over with a spatula. Portion the potatoes and eggs onto individual plates. Top with onion-spinach mixture.

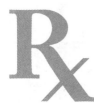

Exchanges/Choices

2 Starch • 2 Vegetable • 1 Med-Fat Meat • 1 1/2 Fat

Calories 350 • Calories from Fat 135 • Total Fat 15.0g • Saturated Fat 3.4g • Trans Fat 0.0g • Cholesterol 315mg • Sodium 155mg • Total Carbohydrate 42g • Dietary Fiber 5g • Sugars 12g • Protein 14g

Salmon, Leek, and Broccoli Quiche

Serves 8 / Serving size: 1/8 recipe

1 recipe	Whole-Wheat Pie Crust

❖ Prepare the crust according to the recipe on p. 27.

1 cup	nonfat milk
3 Tbsp	fat-free sour cream
2 Tbsp	chopped fresh dill
1 Tbsp	black pepper
3	eggs

❖ Preheat oven to 375°F.

❖ In a large bowl, mix milk, sour cream, dill, pepper, and eggs.

10 oz	leeks, trimmed, washed, and cut into 1/4-inch slices
2 cups	broccoli flowerets
8 oz	salmon, sliced

❖ Add leeks, broccoli, and salmon. Pour mixture into pie crust. Bake 35 minutes, until the filling is set and golden.

Exchanges/Choices
1 Starch • 1 Vegetable • 1 Med-Fat Meat • 1/2 Fat

Calories 395 • Calories from Fat 180 • Total Fat 20.0g • Saturated Fat 3.5g • Trans Fat 0.0g • Cholesterol 160mg • Sodium 120mg • Total Carbohydrate 0g • Dietary Fiber 0g • Sugars 0g • Protein 50g

Whole-Wheat Pie Crust

Serves 8 / Serving size: 1/8 recipe

1 1/4 cups	whole-wheat flour
1/4 tsp	salt
1/4 cup	65% buttermilk-vegetable oil spread

❖ Preheat oven to 400°F.

❖ In a large bowl, combine flour and salt. Cut the spread into the flour mixture until the mixture forms coarse crumbs.

2 Tbsp	water

❖ Sprinkle water over mixture, and knead with hands. Use a rolling pin to roll out pastry onto a lightly floured surface to make a 12- to 14-inch circle that is 1/2 inch thick.

❖ To transfer pastry to a pie pan, roll the pastry loosely around the rolling pin. Gently unroll over pie pan. Ease the pastry into the bottom and sides of pan, allowing excess pastry to overhang the edge. Cut off any excess pastry. Using a fork, prick the bottom of the pastry. Cut out a circle of wax paper 3 inches larger than pie pan, and gently press wax paper on the bottom and sides of pastry.

	dry beans or uncooked rice

❖ Fill pastry with dried beans or rice. Bake pastry for 20 minutes. Remove beans and wax paper, and let pie crust cool before filling.

Prescription for Success
The weight of the beans or rice on top of wax or parchment paper allows the crust to cook evenly. This method is called "baking blind." The paper and beans or rice should be removed 5 minutes before baking time is over to allow the crust to brown.

Exchanges/Choices
1 Starch • 1/2 Fat

Calories 0 • Calories from Fat 0 • Total Fat 0.0g • Saturated Fat 0.0g • Trans Fat 0.0g • Cholesterol 0mg • Sodium 0mg • Total Carbohydrate 0g • Dietary Fiber 0g • Sugars 0g • Protein 0g

Asparagus Tips and Tomato Quiche

Serves 8 / Serving size: 1/8 recipe

	nonstick cooking spray
4 oz	turkey bacon

❖ Spray sauté pan with cooking spray, and heat on medium. Cook the turkey bacon, and break into pieces.

❖ Preheat oven to 375°F.

1	small onion, thinly sliced
10 oz	frozen asparagus tips, thawed
4 cloves	garlic
1 cup	nonfat milk
3	large eggs, beaten
1 tsp	black pepper

❖ In large bowl, mix together onion, asparagus, garlic, milk, eggs, and pepper.

1 recipe	Whole-Wheat Pie Crust (p. 27)
4	plum tomatoes, thinly sliced

❖ Pour mixture into pie crust. Top with tomatoes. Bake 35 minutes, until the filling is set and golden.

Exchanges/Choices
1 Starch • 1 Vegetable • 1 Lean Meat • 1/2 Fat

Calories 45 • Calories from Fat 0 • Total Fat 0.0g • Saturated Fat 0.1g • Trans Fat 0.0g • Cholesterol 0mg • Sodium 10mg • Total Carbohydrate 10g • Dietary Fiber 3g • Sugars 7g • Protein 2g

Cranberry Scones

2 cups	all-purpose flour
1 cup	whole-wheat flour
1 1/2 tsp	baking soda
1/2 tsp	salt
1/2 cup	granulated sugar

❖ Preheat oven to 425°F.

❖ In a large bowl, mix flours, baking soda, and salt. Stir in sugar.

8 Tbsp	margarine
1/2 cup	dried cranberries

❖ Cut the margarine into flour mixture until mixture forms coarse crumbs. Stir in cranberries, and make a well in the center.

1	egg
3/4 cup	nonfat milk

❖ Beat the egg and 3/4 cup milk in a small bowl; pour into the well. Stir the flour into the liquid with a fork until it is combined.

❖ Form the dough into a ball, and place on a lightly floured surface. Roll the dough into a 3/4-inch-thick round. To cut rounds, use a 2 1/2-inch wide round cutter. Transfer rounds to a lightly floured baking sheet, arranging them 1 inch apart.

1/4 cup	nonfat milk

❖ Brush the tops with the milk, and bake 15 minutes until golden brown.

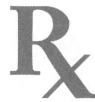

Exchanges/Choices
2 Carbohydrate • 1/2 Fat

Calories 165 • Calories from Fat 40 • Total Fat 4.5g • Saturated Fat 1.2g • Trans Fat 0.0g • Cholesterol 15mg • Sodium 245mg • Total Carbohydrate 28g • Dietary Fiber 2g • Sugars 10g • Protein 4g

Lemon Poppy Muffins

Serves 12 / Serving size: 1 muffin

12	paper cupcake liners

❖ Preheat oven to 425°F, and line muffin pan with cupcake liners.

1 3/4 cups	all-purpose flour
2 Tbsp	granulated sugar
2 tsp	baking powder
1/4 tsp	salt
1 cup	nonfat milk
1/2 tsp	lemon extract
1	egg
1 Tbsp	margarine, melted
2 Tbsp	poppy seeds

❖ Combine all ingredients, and mix until blended. Spoon the batter into the cups, filling each to two-thirds full. Bake 18 minutes, until a toothpick inserted in a muffin comes out clean, and the muffins are golden brown.

Exchanges/Choices
1 Carbohydrate • 1/2 Fat

Calories 100 • Calories from Fat 20 • Total Fat 2.0g • Saturated Fat 0.4g • Trans Fat 0.0g • Cholesterol 20mg • Sodium 130mg • Total Carbohydrate 18g • Dietary Fiber 1g • Sugars 4g • Protein 3g

Challah French Toast with Blueberry Sauce

Serves 6 / Serving size: 1 slice toast

3	large eggs
1 1/2 cups	nonfat milk
1 Tbsp	vanilla extract

❖ In a large bowl, whisk eggs, milk, and vanilla together.

| | nonstick cooking spray |
| 6 1-inch-thick slices | Challah bread |

❖ Lightly spray griddle or heavy skillet with cooking spray, and heat over medium heat. Dip each bread slice into egg mixture, and cook until the tops begin to look dry and the bottoms are golden brown. Turn and brown the other side.

| 1 Tbsp | granulated sugar |
| 1 Tbsp | water |

❖ In a medium saucepan over medium heat, add sugar and water. Cook 3 minutes, until sugar is diluted.

| 1 pint | blueberries, washed |
| 1/2 tsp | lemon juice |

❖ Add blueberries. Continue to cook for 8 minutes, stirring frequently. Stir in lemon juice.

| 2 Tbsp | powdered sugar |

❖ Sprinkle a plate with powdered sugar, top with challah French toast, and spoon warm blueberry sauce on top.

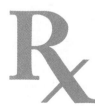

Exchanges/Choices
2 1/2 Starch 1 Fruit 1 Med-Fat Meat

Calories 335 • Calories from Fat 65 • Total Fat 7.0g • Saturated Fat 2.1g • Trans Fat 0.0g • Cholesterol 150mg • Sodium 455mg • Total Carbohydrate 53g • Dietary Fiber 3g • Sugars 14g • Protein 13g

Seared Salmon with Herb Cream Cheese Spread

Serves 4 / Serving size: 1/4 recipe

1 Tbsp	olive oil
4	3-oz salmon fillets
1/4 tsp	salt
1 tsp	pepper

❖ Heat oil in a sauté pan over high heat, season salmon with salt and pepper, and add to pan. Cook 3 minutes on each side, turning once.

4 oz	fat-free cream cheese
4 cloves	garlic, chopped
1 tsp	fresh thyme, chopped
1 tsp	fresh oregano, chopped

❖ Mix all ingredients with an electric mixer. Refrigerate until ready to use.

❖ Top each salmon fillet with 2 Tbsp herb cream cheese spread.

Prescription for Success
Serve with a 2 oz whole-wheat bagel.

Exchanges/Choices
3 Lean Meat • 1 1/2 Fat

Calories 210 • Calories from Fat 100 • Total Fat 11.0g • Saturated Fat 1.8g • Trans Fat 0.0g • Cholesterol 65mg • Sodium 370mg • Total Carbohydrate 3g • Dietary Fiber 0g • Sugars 1g • Protein 23g

Fruited Cottage Cheese Toasts

Serves 8 / Serving size: 1/8 recipe

8 slices	whole-wheat toast

❖ Cut toast into triangles.

4 cups	cubed cantaloupe
1/4 cup	orange juice

❖ In a blender, combine cantaloupe and orange juice.

4 cups	1% cottage cheese

❖ In a bowl, add cantaloupe mixture to cottage cheese. Serve mixture over toast triangles.

Exchanges/Choices
1 Starch • 1/2 Fruit • 2 Lean Meat

Calories 190 • Calories from Fat 20 • Total Fat 2.5g • Saturated Fat 1.0g • Trans Fat 0.0g • Cholesterol 5mg • Sodium 615mg • Total Carbohydrate 23g • Dietary Fiber 3g • Sugars 11g • Protein 19g

Cream Cheese Vegetable Spread

Serves 4 / Serving size: 1/4 recipe

1/4 cup	chopped broccoli

❖ Blanch broccoli by placing it in boiling water for 1 minute, until broccoli turns a vibrant dark-green color. Immediately remove from hot water, and place in ice water.

2 Tbsp	chopped yellow pepper
2 Tbsp	peeled and chopped carrot
1 Tbsp	chopped red onion
4 oz	fat-free cream cheese

❖ Mix broccoli, peppers, carrots, and onion with cream cheese. Serve cold.

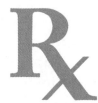

Exchanges/Choices
1/2 Fat-Free Milk

Calories 30 • Calories from Fat 0 • Total Fat 0.0g • Saturated Fat 0.0g • Trans Fat 0.0g • Cholesterol 5mg • Sodium 185mg • Total Carbohydrate 3g • Dietary Fiber 0g • Sugars 1g • Protein 4g

Cinnamon Raisin Quick Bread

1 1/4 cups	all-purpose flour
1 cup	whole-wheat flour
1 1/2 tsp	baking powder
1/2 tsp	baking soda
1/2 tsp	salt
1 tsp	ground cinnamon

❖ Preheat oven to 425°F.

❖ Mix flours, baking powder, baking soda, salt, and cinnamon in a large bowl.

2 cups	low-fat plain yogurt
2	egg whites
1/2 cup	golden raisins
2 Tbsp	honey

❖ Whisk together yogurt and egg whites, and fold into flour mixture with the raisins and honey.

	nonstick cooking spray

❖ Spray a loaf pan with cooking spray. Add mixture to pan, and bake for 25 minutes until golden brown.

Exchanges/Choices
2 Starch • 1 Fruit

Calories 210 • Calories from Fat 15 • Total Fat 1.5g • Saturated Fat 0.7g • Trans Fat 0.0g • Cholesterol 5mg • Sodium 350mg • Total Carbohydrate 42g • Dietary Fiber 3g • Sugars 14g • Protein 8g

Breakfast Burrito

	nonstick cooking spray
1/2 cup	sliced green pepper
1/2 cup	sliced red pepper
1/4 cup	chopped jalapeño pepper
3/4 cup	sliced onion

❖ Spray a sauté pan with cooking spray, and heat on high. Sauté peppers and onions for 3 minutes.

2	4-oz flour tortillas

❖ Meanwhile, preheat the oven to 275°F. Wrap the tortillas in a damp dishtowel, and place in a casserole dish. Cover with a lid or aluminum foil. Heat the tortillas in the oven for 15 minutes or until warm.

1 cup	refried beans

❖ Heat beans in a small pan.

3 oz	reduced-fat sharp cheddar cheese
2 Tbsp	fat-free sour cream

❖ Put beans, peppers, and onions inside tortillas. Top with cheese and sour cream. Fold tortillas, and slice in half diagonally.

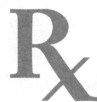

Exchanges/Choices

2 1/2 Starch • 1 Vegetable • 1 Lean Meat • 1/2 Fat

Calories 290 • Calories from Fat 65 • Total Fat 7.0g • Saturated Fat 2.3g • Trans Fat 0.0g • Cholesterol 10mg • Sodium 800mg • Total Carbohydrate 43g • Dietary Fiber 5g • Sugars 4g • Protein 15g

Pimento Herb Omelet

Serves 4 / Serving size: 1/4 recipe

	nonstick cooking spray

❖ Lightly spray a sauté pan with cooking spray, and heat over medium-low heat.

4	large eggs
1/4 cup	chopped pimentos
1 Tbsp	chopped fresh scallions
1 tsp	chopped fresh tarragon
1/4 tsp	salt
1/4 tsp	pepper

❖ In a medium bowl, whisk together eggs, pimentos, scallions, tarragon, salt, and pepper.

1 cup	diced avocado
2 cups	diced tomatoes

❖ Pour mixture into pan; add avocado and tomatoes. Using a spatula, frequently lift edges to allow the uncooked egg to run underneath. Cook for 3 minutes.

2 cups	cubed cantaloupe

❖ Gently fold the omelet in half, and serve with cubed cantaloupe.

Exchanges/Choices
1/2 Fruit • 1 Vegetable • 1 Med-Fat Meat • 1 Fat

Calories 180 • Calories from Fat 100 • Total Fat 11.0g • Saturated Fat 2.4g • Trans Fat 0.0g • Cholesterol 210mg • Sodium 275mg • Total Carbohydrate 15g • Dietary Fiber 5g • Sugars 10g • Protein 9g

Sweet Potato Hash Browns

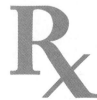

2 cups	*grated sweet potatoes*
1/4 cup	*thinly sliced onion*
1/4 tsp	*salt*
1/2 tsp	*pepper*

❖ In a bowl, combine potatoes, onions, salt, and pepper. Separate mixture into 4 patties.

2 Tbsp	*olive oil*

❖ In a sauté pan, heat oil over medium-high heat, and cook potato mixture for 2 minutes on each side until golden brown.

Exchanges/Choices
1 Starch • 1 Fat

Calories 110 • Calories from Fat 65 • Total Fat 7.0g • Saturated Fat 0.9g • Trans Fat 0.0g • Cholesterol 0mg • Sodium 175mg • Total Carbohydrate 12g • Dietary Fiber 2g • Sugars 3g • Protein 1g

Cheese Blintzes

1	*large egg*
1/4 cup	*all-purpose flour*
1/4 tsp	*sugar*
1/4 cup	*nonfat milk*

❖ In a medium bowl, combine egg, flour, sugar, and milk.

	nonstick cooking spray

❖ Spray a small (5-inch) frying pan with cooking spray, and place over medium heat.

❖ Pour one-fourth of mixture into pan, and circulate pan to coat bottom with batter. Cook 2 minutes, until top looks set and bottom is lightly browned. Flip shells onto a brown paper bag.

4 oz	*1% cottage cheese*
1 1/2 oz	*fat-free cream cheese*
1/4 cup	*confectioner's sugar*
1/2 tsp	*vanilla extract*

❖ Using an electric mixer at medium speed, beat cream cheeses, sugar, and vanilla extract.

❖ Preheat oven to 350°F.

1 Tbsp	*margarine, melted*

❖ Fill each shell with one heaping tablespoon of cheese mixture. Fold sides toward center, and beginning at bottom edge, roll up blintzes. Brush blintzes with melted margarine. Bake for 10 minutes.

Prescription for Success
Serve with fresh seasonal fruit.

Exchanges/Choices
1 Carbohydrate • 1 Lean Meat • 1/2 Fat

Calories 130 • Calories from Fat 30 • Total Fat 3.5g • Saturated Fat 1.1g • Trans Fat 0.0g • Cholesterol 55mg • Sodium 230mg • Total Carbohydrate 16g • Dietary Fiber 0g • Sugars 10g • Protein 8g

Banana Yogurt Oatmeal Loaf

Serves 7 / Serving size: 1 slice

2/3 cup	all-purpose flour
2/3 cup	whole-wheat flour
1/2 cup	instant oatmeal
1 tsp	baking soda
1/4 tsp	salt

❖ Preheat oven to 325°F.

❖ In a medium bowl, combine flours, oatmeal, baking soda, and salt. Set aside.

2 Tbsp	margarine, softened
1/3 cup	brown sugar
1/3 cup	granulated sugar
2	large ripe bananas, mashed
1/2 cup	low-fat vanilla yogurt
2	eggs, lightly beaten
	nonstick cooking spray

❖ In a large bowl, using an electric mixer, beat margarine and sugars until light and fluffy. On low speed, beat in bananas and yogurt. Add the eggs and then the flour mixture.

❖ Spray loaf pan with cooking spray. Add mixture to pan, and bake 1 hour, 15 minutes until dark golden brown.

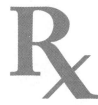

Exchanges/Choices
3 1/2 Carbohydrate • 1 Fat

Calories 270 • Calories from Fat 45 • Total Fat 5.0g • Saturated Fat 1.3g • Trans Fat 0.0g • Cholesterol 60mg • Sodium 340mg • Total Carbohydrate 52g • Dietary Fiber 3g • Sugars 27g • Protein 7g

Cheesy Potato and Spinach Patties

1 1/2 lb	*potatoes*

❖ Boil potatoes in a large pot filled with enough water to cover potatoes by 1 inch. Drain and peel off skin while still warm.

3 oz	*reduced-fat cheddar cheese*
4	*scallions, chopped*
1 cup	*chopped fresh spinach, washed and patted dry*
1 tsp	*pepper*
1	*egg, beaten*

❖ In a large bowl, using an electric mixer, beat potatoes, cheese, scallions, spinach, pepper, and egg. Cover and refrigerate mixture for 1 hour.

1/4 cup	*all-purpose flour*

❖ Divide the mixture into 8 equal patties. Dredge each patty in the flour.

1 Tbsp	*olive oil*

❖ Heat oil in a frying pan. Fry the patties for 2 minutes on each side until golden brown. Drain on paper towels.

Prescription for Success

Serve with a scrambled egg, and top with Mustard Sauce (p. 41).

Exchanges/Choices

1 Starch • 1 Fat

Calories 120 • Calories from Fat 35 • Total Fat 4.0g • Saturated Fat 1.4g • Trans Fat 0.0g • Cholesterol 30mg • Sodium 160mg • Total Carbohydrate 17g • Dietary Fiber 2g • Sugars 1g • Protein 5g

Mustard Sauce

1 tsp	olive oil

❖ Heat oil in sauté pan over medium-high heat.

1 Tbsp	minced shallots
1 tsp	black pepper

❖ Add shallots and pepper; cook for 4 minutes.

1/4 cup	white wine

❖ Add wine. Continue to cook for 10 minutes, until wine has almost completely evaporated. Let cool.

1 Tbsp	Dijon mustard
4 tsp	Creole mustard
1 Tbsp	fat-free mayonnaise
1/4 tsp	honey

❖ Combine shallot-wine mixture with mustards, mayonnaise, and honey. Keep refrigerated.

Prescription for Success

Serve as a warm sauce over cheesy potato and spinach patties.

Exchanges/Choices

Free food

Calories 15 • Calories from Fat 10 • Total Fat 1.0g • Saturated Fat 0.1g • Trans Fat 0.0g • Cholesterol 0mg • Sodium 90mg • Total Carbohydrate 1g • Dietary Fiber 0g • Sugars 1g • Protein 0g

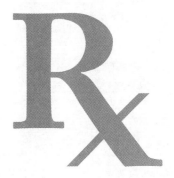

Lunch

Vegetable Goat Cheese Croustades with Mixed Greens Salad

6 slices	7-grain 100% whole-wheat bread

❖ Preheat oven to 400°F.

❖ Place bread slices on a baking sheet and bake for 4 minutes, turning once until lightly toasted.

2 tsp	olive oil
1 cup	sliced Portobello mushrooms
1 cup	chopped red pepper
3 cloves	garlic, chopped
1 tsp	black pepper
2 1/2 oz	soft goat cheese

❖ In sauté pan heat olive oil. Add mushrooms, red peppers, garlic, and black pepper. Sauté for 2 minutes on high heat.

❖ Spoon mixture onto bread croustades, and top with goat cheese. Return to preheated oven for 5 minutes.

9 cups	mixed greens salad
6 Tbsp	balsamic vinaigrette

❖ Toss salad greens with vinaigrette just before serving.

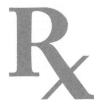

Exchanges/Choices
1 Starch • 1 Vegetable • 1 Fat

Calories 165 • Calories from Fat 55 • Total Fat 6.0g • Saturated Fat 2.2g • Trans Fat 0.0g • Cholesterol 5mg • Sodium 195mg • Total Carbohydrate 21g • Dietary Fiber 4g • Sugars 6g • Protein 8g

Chicken-Stuffed Sweet Potato Skins with Roasted Zucchini and Yogurt Mustard Sauce

Serves 6 / Serving size: 1/6 recipe

1 lb	boneless, skinless chicken breast

❖ Preheat grill and cook chicken until done. Set aside to cool. When cool enough to handle, cut into slices.

1 1/2 lb	sweet potatoes

❖ Preheat oven to 350°F.

❖ Bake sweet potatoes for 30 minutes. Slice potatoes in half lengthwise, and scoop out potato centers, leaving a thick border around the skin. Set scooped potato aside in a large bowl. Add sliced chicken to potato skins.

2 tsp	hot sauce
4 cloves	garlic

❖ Combine hot sauce, garlic, and scooped potatoes. Spoon mixture on top of chicken. Place potato skins on a baking pan. Bake at 350°F for 10 minutes.

1 lb	whole zucchini, sliced lengthwise
2 tsp	olive oil
1 tsp	black pepper

❖ Coat zucchini with olive oil, season with black pepper, and roast in the oven for 10 minutes.

4 oz	low-fat plain yogurt
1 Tbsp	yellow mustard

❖ Mix yogurt and mustard. Spoon the mixture over chicken, and serve the zucchini on the side.

Exchanges/Choices
1 Starch • 1 Vegetable • 3 Lean Meat

Calories 250 • Calories from Fat 45 • Total Fat 5.0g • Saturated Fat 1.2g • Trans Fat 0.0g • Cholesterol 65mg • Sodium 150mg • Total Carbohydrate 24g • Dietary Fiber 4g • Sugars 9g • Protein 27g

Veggie Pita Pizza

| 2 | pitas, sliced lengthwise |

❖ Toast pitas on a cookie sheet in a preheated 300°F oven for 6 minutes or until golden brown.

1 1/2 Tbsp	olive oil
1/4 cup	mushrooms, thick sliced
1/4 cup	zucchini, thick sliced
1/4 cup	yellow squash, thick sliced
1/4 cup	onion, sliced thin
1/4 cup	red pepper, cut into strips
12	cherry tomatoes, sliced in half
12 cloves	garlic
12 oz	fresh baby spinach

❖ Over high heat in a large sauté pan, heat oil. Add mushrooms, zucchini, squash, onions, and red pepper; cook for 2 minutes. Add tomatoes, garlic, and spinach, and cook until spinach is wilted.

| 1 1/2 oz | freshly grated Parmesan cheese |

❖ Remove pitas from oven, spread vegetable mixture on pitas, and top with cheese. Return pita pizzas to the oven for 4 minutes. Plate each pita, and cut into four slices.

Prescription for Success

The choice of vegetables—broccoli, red onion, yellow and orange peppers— are wonderfully endless! Color and variety are key components to making a healthy meal you will want to have over and over again.

Exchanges/Choices

1 Starch • 2 Vegetable • 1 Med-Fat Meat • 1/2 Fat

Calories 215 • Calories from Fat 80 • Total Fat 9.0g • Saturated Fat 2.4g • Trans Fat 0.0g • Cholesterol 10mg • Sodium 300mg • Total Carbohydrate 26g • Dietary Fiber 4g • Sugars 3g • Protein 10g

Vegetarian Chili

Serves 4 / Serving size: 1/4 recipe

1 Tbsp	olive oil

❖ Heat olive oil in large pot over medium heat.

1/4 cup	diced onions
1/4 cup	diced celery
1/4 cup	diced green pepper
1/4 cup	diced carrots

❖ Add onions, celery, green pepper, and carrots. Cook and stir for 4 minutes.

4 cloves	garlic, chopped
2 Tbsp	chili powder
1 tsp	ground cumin
15.5-oz can	lentils, drained
6	plum tomatoes, concassé
1/2 cup	unsweetened pineapple juice
1/2 cup	tomato-based chili sauce
2 Tbsp	molasses

❖ Add garlic, chili powder, cumin, lentils, tomatoes, pineapple juice, chili sauce, and molasses. Cover and simmer for 20 minutes, stirring occasionally. Remove from heat.

4 tsp	low-fat sour cream
1/4 cup	chopped fresh cilantro

❖ Ladle into four serving bowls, and top each with 1 tsp sour cream and cilantro.

Prescription for Success

Concassé means to roughly chop or cut. Here is how to prepare tomato concassé. Bring a pot of water to a boil. Cut an X into the bottom of each tomato. Drop the tomatoes into the water for 15 seconds. Remove with a slotted spoon, and immediately place tomatoes in a bowl of ice water. Pull away the skin, cut the tomatoes lengthwise, and gently squeeze out the seeds. Cut the tomatoes into chunks.

Exchanges/Choices

1/2 Carbohydrate • 3 Vegetable

Calories 250 • Calories from Fat 45 • Total Fat 5.0g • Saturated Fat 1.0g • Trans Fat 0.0g • Cholesterol 0mg • Sodium 565mg • Total Carbohydrate 42g • Dietary Fiber 11g • Sugars 18g • Protein 10g

Beef with Broccoli

Serves 4 / Serving size: 1/4 recipe

1 Tbsp	olive oil
1	small red pepper, chopped
2	scallions, chopped
4 cloves	garlic, chopped
2 Tbsp	soy sauce

❖ In a wok or sauté pan, heat oil. Add red pepper, scallions, garlic, and soy sauce. Cook for 2 minutes.

3/4 lb	lean flank steak, thinly sliced
1 1/2 cups	broccoli florets

❖ Add steak and broccoli, and cook for 5 minutes, stirring occasionally.

1 1/3 cups	cooked rice

❖ Divide rice among four bowls. Top with beef and broccoli mixture.

Prescription for Success
This dish can be spiced up with any of a variety of hot spices, such as cayenne pepper, chili powder, chipotle pepper, or Tabasco sauce.

Exchanges/Choices
1 Starch • 1 Vegetable • 2 Lean Meat • 1 Fat

Calories 235 • Calories from Fat 70 • Total Fat 8.0g • Saturated Fat 2.4g • Trans Fat 0.0g • Cholesterol 30mg • Sodium 495mg • Total Carbohydrate 20g • Dietary Fiber 2g • Sugars 2g • Protein 20g

Turkey-Veggie Burger

Serves 4 / Serving size: 1 patty

3/4 lb	lean ground turkey
1/4 cup	frozen peas
1/4 cup	shredded carrots
1/4 cup	chopped mushrooms
2	eggs, lightly beaten

❖ In a large bowl, combine turkey, peas, carrots, mushrooms, and eggs. Divide mixture into four patties.

	nonstick cooking spray

❖ Spray a skillet with cooking spray, and heat on medium heat. Cook patties for 4 minutes on one side; then turn over and cook for an additional 3 minutes.

4	whole-wheat hamburger buns
1 cup	shredded iceberg lettuce
4	medium slices tomato
4	medium slices red onion

❖ Place a burger on each roll. Top with lettuce, tomato, and onion.

3 cups	cubed cantaloupe

❖ Serve with a side of cantaloupe.

Prescription for Success
Any mixture of your favorite vegetables may be used. The patties will be easier to handle if the vegetables are cut into smaller pieces.

Exchanges/Choices
2 Starch • 1/2 Fruit • 3 Lean Meat

Calories 340 • Calories from Fat 100 • Total Fat 11.0g • Saturated Fat 3.1g • Trans Fat 0.0g • Cholesterol 165mg • Sodium 330mg • Total Carbohydrate 36g • Dietary Fiber 6g • Sugars 15g • Protein 26g

Spicy Flounder Sandwich

1	medium onion, chopped
4 cloves	garlic, chopped
8-oz can	no-added-salt tomato sauce
1 1/2 tsp	hot sauce
1 tsp	Worcestershire sauce

❖ In a large skillet over medium heat, cook onion, garlic, tomato sauce, hot sauce, and Worcestershire sauce.

3/4 lb	flounder fillet, cut into large chunks

❖ Top mixture with fish chunks. Cook for 5 minutes, until fish flakes easily with a fork.

4	whole-wheat hamburger buns
1 cup	chopped lettuce
4 slices	tomato
4 slices	red onion

❖ Spoon mixture onto rolls, and top with lettuce, tomato, and onion.

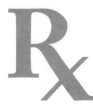

Exchanges/Choices

1 1/2 Starch • 2 Vegetable • 2 Lean Meat

Calories 240 • Calories from Fat 30 • Total Fat 3.5g • Saturated Fat 0.6g • Trans Fat 0.0g • Cholesterol 45mg • Sodium 325mg • Total Carbohydrate 34g • Dietary Fiber 6g • Sugars 9g • Protein 22g

Chicken Souvlaki with Tzatziki Sauce

Serves 4 / Serving size: 1 pita

4	small (4-inch) whole-wheat pitas

❖ Wrap pitas in foil, and warm them in a preheated 200°F oven.

1 Tbsp	olive oil
1 Tbsp	red wine vinegar
1 tsp	lemon juice

❖ In a small bowl, combine 1 Tbsp oil, vinegar, and lemon juice.

2	vine-ripened tomatoes, cut into wedges
1	small red onion, thinly sliced
2 oz	reduced-fat feta cheese

❖ In a separate bowl, combine tomatoes, onion, and feta cheese. Add oil mixture, and toss to coat.

1 Tbsp	chopped fresh oregano
1 Tbsp	chopped fresh thyme
1/4 tsp	pepper
1 Tbsp	olive oil
3/4 lb	boneless, skinless chicken breasts, cut into pieces

❖ In a large bowl, combine oregano, thyme, pepper, and olive oil. Add chicken, and toss until well coated. Over medium-high heat, add chicken mixture to a hot skillet. Cook chicken for 5 minutes, turning frequently to cook evenly.

1/2 cup	fat-free plain yogurt
1	small cucumber, peeled and diced
1 Tbsp	chopped fresh dill

❖ Meanwhile, in a small bowl, combine yogurt, cucumber, and dill. Spread sauce on warm pitas, top with chicken, and then top with tomato mixture.

Exchanges/Choices
1 Starch • 1 Vegetable • 3 Lean Meat • 1 1/2 Fat

Calories 305 • Calories from Fat 110 • Total Fat 12.0g • Saturated Fat 2.9g • Trans Fat 0.0g • Cholesterol 55mg • Sodium 410mg • Total Carbohydrate 24g • Dietary Fiber 4g • Sugars 5g • Protein 26g

Grilled Turkey Panini

1/2 oz	turkey bacon

❖ Cook bacon in a skillet over medium heat.

	nonstick cooking spray
3/4 lb	skinless, boneless turkey breast

❖ Heat grill and spray with cooking spray. Grill turkey cutlet for 4 minutes on each side until fully cooked. When it is cool enough to handle, slice thinly.

8 slices	whole-wheat bread
4 Tbsp	fat-free mayonnaise
1 cup	shredded iceberg lettuce
4	medium tomato slices

❖ Lightly grill each slice of bread. Spread mayonnaise over 4 slices of bread. Portion the turkey over the remaining 4 slices of bread, and top with bacon, lettuce, and tomato.

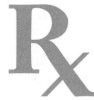

Exchanges/Choices
2 Starch • 2 Lean Meat

Calories 255 • Calories from Fat 30 • Total Fat 3.5g • Saturated Fat 0.8g • Trans Fat 0.5g • Cholesterol 60mg • Sodium 465mg • Total Carbohydrate 26g • Dietary Fiber 5g • Sugars 5g • Protein 28g

Pasta Primavera in a Light Béchamel Sauce

Serves 4 / Serving size: 1/4 recipe

1/2 lb	whole-wheat linguini pasta

❖ Cook pasta in a large pot of boiling water until al dente. Drain water.

1 Tbsp	olive oil
1/2 cup	sliced onion
1/2 cup	cut broccoli
1/4 cup	sliced zucchini
1/4 cup	sliced yellow squash
1/4 cup	sliced mushrooms
1/4 cup	sliced red pepper

❖ Meanwhile, heat oil in a sauté pan on medium-high heat, add onion, broccoli, zucchini, squash, mushrooms, and red pepper. Cook for 3 minutes.

1 Tbsp	margarine
1 Tbsp	all-purpose flour

❖ Combine margarine and flour to make a roux. Cook in a medium saucepan over low heat for 5 minutes.

1 cup	nonfat milk
1/2 tsp	salt
1/2 tsp	pepper
1/2 tsp	garlic powder
1/2 tsp	onion powder

❖ To roux, add milk, salt, pepper, and garlic and onion powders. Cook for 5 minutes, until sauce is smooth.

2 Tbsp	fresh cut parsley

❖ Combine pasta, vegetables, and sauce; top with fresh parsley.

Exchanges/Choices
3 Starch • 1 Fat

Calories 300 • Calories from Fat 65 • Total Fat 7.0g • Saturated Fat 1.2g • Trans Fat 0.0g • Cholesterol 0mg • Sodium 350mg • Total Carbohydrate 49g • Dietary Fiber 7g • Sugars 6g • Protein 12g

Shrimp Ratatouille

2 Tbsp	olive oil
1/2 cup	onions, diced
1/2 cup	eggplant, diced
1/2 cup	yellow peppers, diced
1/2 cup	zucchini, diced
1	8-oz can artichoke hearts, diced

❖ In a skillet over medium-high heat, add oil, onions, eggplant, peppers, zucchini, and artichoke hearts. Cook for 2 minutes.

1/4 cup	low-sodium chicken broth
6 cloves	garlic, chopped
1/2 cup	cherry tomatoes
1/4 tsp	dried marjoram
1/4 tsp	dried basil
3/4 lb	peeled and cleaned large shrimp

❖ Add broth, garlic, tomatoes, marjoram, basil, and shrimp. Cook 3 more minutes, until shrimp turns pink.

4 slices	French bread, toasted

❖ Equally divide mixture over toasted bread.

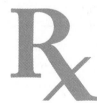

Exchanges/Choices

1 Starch • 2 Vegetable • 2 Lean Meat • 1 Fat

Calories 265 • Calories from Fat 70 • Total Fat 8.0g • Saturated Fat 1.4g • Trans Fat 0.0g • Cholesterol 120mg • Sodium 500mg • Total Carbohydrate 29g • Dietary Fiber 4g • Sugars 4g • Protein 19g

Tuna Wrap

Serves 4 / Serving size: 1 wrap

2	6-oz cans white albacore tuna packed in water, drained
1/2 cup	minced onion
1/4 cup	finely chopped celery
1/2 tsp	pepper
1/2 cup	fat-free mayonnaise

❖ Combine tuna, onion, celery, pepper, and mayonnaise; mix well.

2	8-inch tortillas
1 cup	shredded lettuce
1	large tomato, sliced thin

❖ Spread mixture evenly over tortillas. Cover with lettuce and tomato. Roll tortillas, and slice diagonally in the center.

Exchanges/Choices
1 Starch • 1 Vegetable • 2 Lean Meat

Calories 205 • Calories from Fat 45 • Total Fat 5.0g • Saturated Fat 1.2g • Trans Fat 0.0g • Cholesterol 35mg • Sodium 640mg • Total Carbohydrate 20g • Dietary Fiber 3g • Sugars 5g • Protein 20g

Chicken Cheddar Hoagie

	nonstick cooking spray

❖ Over medium-high heat, lightly spray a large skillet with cooking spray.

1	medium onion, sliced thin
4 cloves	garlic, chopped
1	green pepper, sliced thin

❖ Cook onion, garlic, and peppers, stirring frequently for 3 minutes.

1 Tbsp	olive oil
3/4 lb	chicken breast, thinly sliced

❖ Meanwhile, in a separate skillet, heat the oil. Add chicken, and cook for 2 minutes, turning to cook both sides.

4	5-inch hoagie rolls, toasted
2 oz	reduced-fat cheddar cheese

❖ Stir chicken into the vegetables, place onto toasted hoagie rolls, and top with cheese.

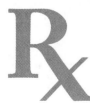

Exchanges/Choices
2 Starch • 1 Vegetable • 3 Lean Meat • 1/2 Fat

Calories 330 • Calories from Fat 70 • Total Fat 8.0g • Saturated Fat 2.4g • Trans Fat 0.0g • Cholesterol 55mg • Sodium 445mg • Total Carbohydrate 36g • Dietary Fiber 2g • Sugars 5g • Protein 28g

Tuna Casserole

1/2 lb	whole-wheat penne pasta

❖ Preheat oven to 350°F.

❖ Cook pasta in a large pot of boiling water until al dente. Drain water.

1 Tbsp	margarine
1 Tbsp	all-purpose flour

❖ Combine margarine and flour to make a roux. Cook in a medium saucepan over low heat for 5 minutes.

1 cup	nonfat milk
1/2 tsp	pepper
1 oz	Parmesan cheese

❖ To roux, add milk, pepper, and cheese. Cook for 5 minutes, until sauce is smooth.

1	6-oz can water-packed white albacore tuna, drained
1 tsp	paprika

❖ Combine pasta, tuna, and sauce in a casserole dish. Sprinkle with paprika, and bake for 20 minutes.

Exchanges/Choices
3 Starch • 2 Lean Meat • 1/2 Fat

Calories 345 • Calories from Fat 55 • Total Fat 6.0g • Saturated Fat 2.4g • Trans Fat 0.0g • Cholesterol 25mg • Sodium 295mg • Total Carbohydrate 50g • Dietary Fiber 6g • Sugars 5g • Protein 21g

Stuffed Eggplant with Rice

2 Tbsp	margarine
1/2 cup	white rice
1/2 cup	brown rice
1	onion, minced
1/2 cup	chopped celery
1/2 cup	chopped carrots
6 cloves	garlic, chopped
1 1/2 cups	low-sodium chicken broth
1 cup	water

❖ Preheat oven to 350°F.

❖ In a medium saucepan over medium heat, melt margarine. Add white and brown rice. Cook for 1 minute, stirring frequently. Reduce heat to low. Add onion, celery, carrots, garlic, broth, and water. Cover and let simmer for 15 minutes or until all water is absorbed.

2	large eggplants, halved lengthwise
	nonstick cooking spray

❖ Scoop out center of eggplants, discarding seeds. Place eggplants on a shallow baking pan coated with cooking spray. Stuff rice mixture into eggplants, and roast in the oven for 15 minutes.

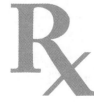

Exchanges/Choices
2 1/2 Starch • 4 Vegetable • 1/2 Fat

Calories 320 • Calories from Fat 55 • Total Fat 6.0g • Saturated Fat 1.4g • Trans Fat 0.0g • Cholesterol 0mg • Sodium 110mg • Total Carbohydrate 63g • Dietary Fiber 8g • Sugars 10g • Protein 7g

Steak Fajitas

Serves 4 / Serving size: 1/4 recipe

1/2 Tbsp	olive oil
2 Tbsp	lime juice
1 Tbsp	chopped red pepper
4 cloves	garlic, chopped
3/4 lb	lean skirt steak, thinly sliced

❖ Combine 1/2 Tbsp oil with lime juice, red pepper, and garlic; mix well. Add steak to marinade, and refrigerate for 3 hours or overnight.

❖ With a slotted spoon, remove steak from marinade.

❖ In a small pan, heat the marinade.

1/2 Tbsp	olive oil
1	large onion, sliced thin
1	medium green pepper, sliced

❖ Cook steak in olive oil in a large sauté pan over high heat for 2 minutes. Add onion and green pepper; cook for 2 minutes more. Add heated marinade.

4	6-inch tortillas
4 Tbsp	fat-free sour cream
1/2 cup	fat-free refried beans, heated
1/2 cup	salsa

❖ Place steak mixture in tortillas. Serve with sour cream, refried beans, and salsa.

Exchanges/Choices
1 1/2 Starch • 2 Vegetable • 2 Lean Meat • 2 Fat

Calories 345 • Calories from Fat 135 • Total Fat 15.0g • Saturated Fat 4.8g • Trans Fat 0.0g • Cholesterol 35mg • Sodium 595mg • Total Carbohydrate 33g • Dietary Fiber 5g • Sugars 6g • Protein 21g

Pulled Pork Sandwich

Serves 4 / Serving size: 1 sandwich

3/4 lb	boneless lean pork loin

❖ Place pork in a small saucepan, cover with water, and cook over low heat for 1 1/2 hours, until fully cooked.

	nonstick cooking spray
1	small onion, minced
3	garlic cloves, minced
1	jalapeño pepper, minced

❖ Spray a sauté pan with cooking spray, and place over high heat. Cook onion, garlic, and jalapeño for 2 minutes.

1/2 cup	low-sodium chicken broth
1/4 cup	ketchup
6 oz	low-sodium tomato juice
1 Tbsp	Worcestershire sauce
1 Tbsp	white vinegar
2 Tbsp	brown sugar
1 tsp	lemon juice
1 tsp	orange juice
3 Tbsp	Dijon mustard

❖ Transfer onion-garlic mixture to a large saucepan over low heat. Add broth, ketchup, tomato juice, Worcestershire sauce, vinegar, sugar, juices, and mustard. Let simmer 20 minutes, stirring frequently.

4	whole-wheat hamburger buns

❖ Remove pork when done, and pull meat into strips. Add pork to mixture; stir to coat well. Spoon pork mixture onto buns.

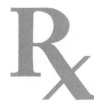

Exchanges/Choices
2 Starch • 2 Vegetable • 2 Lean Meat • 1/2 Fat

Calories 315 • Calories from Fat 70 • Total Fat 8.0g • Saturated Fat 2.3g • Trans Fat 0.0g • Cholesterol 45mg • Sodium 740mg • Total Carbohydrate 42g • Dietary Fiber 4g • Sugars 18g • Protein 22g

Cajun Chicken Kabob

Serves 4 / Serving size: 1 kabob

6 cloves	garlic, minced
1	small onion, minced
2 tsp	chili powder
1/2 tsp	black pepper
2 tsp	Dijon mustard
1 tsp	celery seed
2 Tbsp	oil

❖ Combine garlic, minced onion, chili powder, black pepper, mustard, celery seed, and oil; mix well.

3/4 lb	boneless, skinless chicken breast

❖ Cut chicken into large cubes, add to marinade, and toss to coat.

1	small onion, cut into large cubes
1	red pepper, cut into large cubes

❖ Thread cubed chicken, onion cubes, and pepper cubes onto skewers.

	nonstick cooking spray

❖ Heat the grill on medium, and spray with cooking spray.

1 cup	cooked white rice

❖ Place kabobs on grill, and brush with marinade. Grill chicken kabobs 2 minutes on each side, until fully cooked. Serve over rice.

Prescription for Success
- To prevent burning, soak wooden skewers in water for 20 minutes prior to use.
- Discard any marinade that has not been properly cooked.

Exchanges/Choices
1 Starch • 1 Vegetable • 2 Lean Meat • 1 Fat

Calories 255 • Calories from Fat 90 • Total Fat 10.0 g • Saturated Fat 1.7g • Trans Fat 0.0g • Cholesterol 50mg • Sodium 120mg • Total Carbohydrate 21g • Dietary Fiber 3g • Sugars 4g • Protein 21g

Focaccia Pizza

Serves 8 / Serving size: 1 slice

20 oz	bread flour
1 tsp	salt
2 cups	water, room temperature
1/2 tsp	yeast

❖ Preheat oven to 400°F.

❖ Combine flour and salt. Place flour on a large, clean surface. Make a well in the center of the flour. To center, add water and yeast; let dissolve. Mix ingredients until dough is smooth and elastic.

	nonstick cooking spray

❖ Place dough in a container lightly sprayed with nonstick cooking spray, cover, and let rise for 1 hour, 15 minutes until doubled in volume.

❖ Punch down dough once, and shape into a rough rectangle. Let relax until workable. Spray a sheet pan with cooking spray. Place the dough in pan; score the top.

1 Tbsp	olive oil
8 cloves	garlic, chopped
2 tsp	fresh chopped thyme
2 tsp	fresh chopped oregano
1	small onion, thinly sliced
3	medium vine-ripened tomatoes, thinly sliced
6 oz	part-skim shredded mozzarella cheese

❖ Brush dough with olive oil. Spread with garlic, thyme, oregano, onion, tomatoes, and mozzarella.

❖ Bake at 400°F for 30 minutes, until golden brown.

Exchanges/Choices
3 1/2 Starch • 1 Vegetable • 1 Med-Fat Meat

Calories 345 • Calories from Fat 55 • Total Fat 6.0g • Saturated Fat 2.4g • Trans Fat 0.0g • Cholesterol 15mg • Sodium 430mg • Total Carbohydrate 56g • Dietary Fiber 3g • Sugars 2g • Protein 14g

R_X

Soups

Cajun Fish Soup

2 Tbsp	olive oil
4	green onions, chopped
4 cloves	garlic, minced
2 stalks	celery, chopped
1	green pepper, chopped
1 tsp	paprika
1 tsp	dried thyme leaves
1/2 tsp	cayenne pepper

❖ In a large saucepan, heat oil over medium heat. Add green onions, garlic, celery, green pepper, paprika, thyme, and cayenne pepper. Cook, stirring, for 2 minutes.

2 cups	potatoes, peeled and diced
2	8-oz cans low-sodium stewed diced tomatoes
2 cups	low-sodium vegetable broth

❖ Add potatoes, tomatoes, and broth. Bring to a boil, reduce heat, cover, and simmer for 20 minutes.

1 Tbsp	black pepper
1 Tbsp	Cajun spice
1 lb	firm white fish fillets

❖ Stir in black pepper and Cajun spice. Add fish fillets. Simmer for 2 minutes or until fish flakes when tested with a fork.

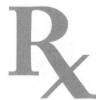

Exchanges/Choices
1 Starch • 3 Vegetable • 3 Lean Meat • 1 1/2 Fat

Calories 360 • Calories from Fat 125 • Total Fat 14.0g • Saturated Fat 2.1g • Trans Fat 0.0g • Cholesterol 70mg • Sodium 405mg • Total Carbohydrate 32g • Dietary Fiber 6g • Sugars 9g • Protein 26g

Five Onion Soup

1 Tbsp	olive oil
2 cups	sliced Vidalia onions
1 cup	sliced leeks
1/2 cup	sliced scallions
1/2 cup	chopped shallots

❖ In a large sauté pan, heat oil. Add onions, leeks, scallions, and shallots. Cook over low heat for 15 minutes, until onions caramelize.

31 oz	fat-free, low-sodium beef broth
1 Tbsp	black pepper

❖ In a large stockpot, add broth, caramelized onions, and pepper. Bring to a boil, lower heat, and simmer for 20 minutes.

4	baguette slices, toasted, about 1/2 oz each
4 tsp	chopped chives

❖ Ladle soup into bowls, add one toasted baguette to each bowl, and top with chives. Serve hot.

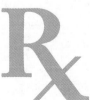

Exchanges/Choices
1/2 Starch • 3 Vegetable • 1/2 Fat

Calories 140 • Calories from Fat 35 • Total Fat 4.0g • Saturated Fat 0.6g • Trans Fat 0.0g • Cholesterol 0mg • Sodium 225mg • Total Carbohydrate 22g • Dietary Fiber 3g • Sugars 5g • Protein 6g

Big Easy Gumbo

1/4 cup	all-purpose flour
1/4 cup	margarine

❖ Combine flour and margarine by hand until well mixed. In a large heavy saucepan, cook mixture over low heat for 15 minutes, stirring constantly.

1/4 cup	chopped onions
1/4 cup	chopped red pepper
1/4 cup	chopped green pepper
6 cloves	garlic, minced
1/2 tsp	ground red pepper
1 tsp	Cajun spice

❖ Stir in onions, red pepper, green pepper, garlic, ground red pepper, and Cajun spice.

2 1/2 cups	low-sodium chicken broth
8 oz	tomato sauce
1	jalapeño, seeded and minced
5 oz	frozen cut okra
2	bay leaves

❖ Gradually stir in chicken broth. Stir in tomato sauce, jalapeño, okra, and bay leaves. Cover and simmer for 40 minutes.

1/2 lb	fresh shrimp, peeled and deveined
1/2 lb	fresh crabmeat

❖ Stir in shrimp and crabmeat. Continue cooking for 5 minutes. Discard bay leaves.

1 cup	cooked rice

❖ Divide rice into 4 bowls, top with gumbo, and serve hot.

Prescription for Success

A mixture of flour and fat is called a "roux" and is used to thicken soups and sauces. Roux is slowly cooked over low heat. The color and flavor are determined by the length of time it is cooked. Three classic types of roux include white, blond, and brown. The darker roux is used for rich, dark soups and sauces such as gumbo.

Exchanges/Choices
1 Starch • 2 Vegetable • 3 Lean Meat • 1 Fat

Calories 295 • Calories from Fat 90 • Total Fat 10.0g • Saturated Fat 2.5g • Trans Fat 0.0g • Cholesterol 130mg • Sodium 740mg • Total Carbohydrate 28g • Dietary Fiber 3g • Sugars 5g • Protein 24g

Vegetable Pesto Soup

2 tsp	olive oil

❖ In a large saucepan over medium heat, heat the oil.

2	onions, chopped

❖ Add onions, and cook 8 minutes, until tender.

2	carrots, peeled and sliced
2	celery stalks, chopped

❖ Add the carrots and celery. Cook for 2 minutes.

1	large tomato, peeled, seeded and chopped
2 cups	low-sodium chicken broth
2 cup	water
1 tsp	black pepper
1/2 cup	cooked navy beans
1/2 cup	cut green beans
1/2 cup	cut zucchini
2 oz	small whole-wheat pasta shells

❖ Add the tomato, broth, water, pepper, navy beans, green beans, zucchini, and pasta. Simmer for 25 minutes, uncovered.

3 cloves	garlic
1/3 cup	fresh basil leaves
2 Tbsp	reduced-fat Parmesan cheese
2 tsp	olive oil

❖ In a food processor or blender, add garlic, basil, and Parmesan cheese. Gradually add oil, and process until mixture forms a coarse texture. Do not overprocess.

❖ Divide soup into serving bowls, and stir in pesto mixture.

Exchanges/Choices
1 Starch • 3 Vegetable • 1 Fat

Calories 210 • Calories from Fat 55 • Total Fat 6.0g • Saturated Fat 1.2g • Trans Fat 0.0g • Cholesterol 5mg • Sodium 160mg • Total Carbohydrate 34g • Dietary Fiber 7g • Sugars 8g • Protein 8g

Hearty Roasted Vegetable Soup

Serves 6 / Serving size: 1/6 recipe

2 1/2 cups	low-sodium chicken broth
3 cups	water
1/4 tsp	dried oregano
1/4 tsp	dried thyme
1 tsp	pepper

❖ Heat oven to 350°F.

❖ In a large saucepan, heat the broth, water, oregano, thyme, and pepper.

2	medium potatoes, cut into equally large chunks
1	small red onion, sliced
1/2 cup	green beans
1/2 cup	red pepper, chopped
1/2 cup	zucchini, sliced
1/4 cup	carrots, chopped
1/4 cup	celery, chopped
6 cloves	garlic, chopped
3 Tbsp	olive oil

❖ In a large bowl, combine potatoes, onion, green beans, red pepper, zucchini, carrots, celery, and garlic. Drizzle olive oil over ingredients, and mix to coat. Spread vegetables onto a baking pan. Roast in preheated oven for 10 minutes.

1/2 cup	cherry tomatoes

❖ Turn vegetables over, add cherry tomatoes, and roast for 5 more minutes.

❖ Carefully add vegetables to broth. Let simmer for 15 minutes. Serve hot.

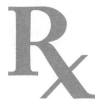

Exchanges/Choices
1 Starch • 1 Vegetable • 1 Fat

Calories 145 • Calories from Fat 65 • Total Fat 7.0g • Saturated Fat 1.0g • Trans Fat 0.0g • Cholesterol 0mg • Sodium 55mg • Total Carbohydrate 18g • Dietary Fiber 3g • Sugars 3g • Protein 3g

Minestrone Soup

1 Tbsp	olive oil
1/2 cup	onion, chopped
1/4 cup	diced celery
1/4 cup	diced carrots
1/4 cup	diced green peppers
1/4 cup	cut green cabbage
4 cloves	garlic

❖ In a large pot, heat oil. Add onions, celery, carrots, green pepper, cabbage, and garlic. Cook for 5 minutes.

2	tomatoes, concassé
1 1/2 cups	low-sodium chicken broth
2 1/2 cups	water
1/2 tsp	pepper

❖ Add tomatoes, broth, water, and pepper. Simmer for 25 minutes.

2 oz	cooked black-eyed peas
2 oz	whole-wheat pasta

❖ Add peas and pasta. Simmer for 15 minutes.

Prescription for Success

Tomato concassé is a tomato that has been peeled and seeded. We do this by scoring an ✕ on the bottom of the tomato with a knife. Place the tomato in boiling water for 1 minute and quickly put into a bowl of ice water to prevent further cooking. The tomato skin will easily peel off. Slice the tomato and remove the seeds.

Exchanges/Choices
1 Starch • 2 Vegetable • 1 Fat

Calories 165 • Calories from Fat 35 • Total Fat 4.0g • Saturated Fat 0.7g • Trans Fat 0.0g • Cholesterol 0mg • Sodium 60mg • Total Carbohydrate 26g • Dietary Fiber 6g • Sugars 5g • Protein 7g

Lentil Soup

1 Tbsp	olive oil
1	large onion, chopped
1	carrot, chopped
1	celery stalk, chopped

❖ In a large pot, heat oil. Add the onions, carrot, and celery. Sauté for 10 minutes, until tender and light golden brown.

1 1/2 cups	low-sodium chicken broth
4 1/2 cups	water
1 cup	dried lentils

❖ Add broth, water, and lentils; bring to a boil. Reduce heat to low, cover, and simmer 40 minutes, until lentils are soft.

1/2 tsp	ground cumin
1/4 tsp	nutmeg

❖ Add cumin and nutmeg; mix well. Purée soup in a blender.

2 tsp	lemon juice
1/4 tsp	salt
1/2 tsp	pepper

❖ Reheat soup, and season with lemon juice, salt, and pepper.

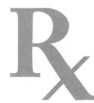

Exchanges/Choices
2 Starch • 1 Vegetable • 1 Lean Meat

Calories 220 • Calories from Fat 35 • Total Fat 4.0g • Saturated Fat 0.7g • Trans Fat 0.0g • Cholesterol 0mg • Sodium 215mg • Total Carbohydrate 34g • Dietary Fiber 12g • Sugars 6g • Protein 14g

Cream of Tomato Soup

Serves 4 / Serving size: 1/4 recipe

2 Tbsp	all-purpose flour
1 Tbsp	margarine

❖ In a bowl, combine flour and margarine to prepare a roux. In a large stockpot, cook roux over low heat, stirring constantly for 10 minutes.

1 Tbsp	olive oil
1/4 cup	chopped carrots
1/4 cup	chopped celery
1/4 cup	chopped onions
2 cloves	garlic, minced

❖ In a separate pot, heat oil. Add carrots, celery, onions, and garlic. Sauté for 10 minutes.

16 oz	tomato purée
1 cup	low-sodium chicken broth
1 tsp	pepper
1	bay leaf

❖ To the stockpot, add vegetable mixture, tomato purée, broth, pepper, and bay leaf. Stir well, and simmer for 30 minutes.

1/4 cup	2% reduced-fat milk
2	sprigs parsley, chopped

❖ Strain soup, and return drained liquid to pot over low heat. Gradually stir in the milk and parsley.

Exchanges/Choices
3 Vegetable (or 1 Carbohydrate) • 1 Fat

Calories 120 • Calories from Fat 55 • Total Fat 6.0g • Saturated Fat 1.3g • Trans Fat 0.0g • Cholesterol 0mg • Sodium 505mg • Total Carbohydrate 15g • Dietary Fiber 3g • Sugars 7g • Protein 4g

Chicken Noodle Soup

1 lb	*boneless, skinless chicken breasts, cubed*
3 cups	*low-sodium chicken broth*
2 cups	*water*
1/2 cup	*chopped onion*
1/2 cup	*sliced carrots*
1/2 cup	*sliced celery*
1	*small turnip, cubed*
1 tsp	*pepper*

❖ In a large pot, add all ingredients. Simmer for 40 minutes, skimming the top as necessary.

2 Tbsp	*chopped fresh dill*
1 cup	*uncooked noodles*

❖ Stir in the dill and noodles, and cook for 10 minutes, until noodles are al dente.

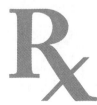

Exchanges/Choices
1/2 Starch • 1 Lean Meat

Calories 100 • Calories from Fat 20 • Total Fat 2.0g • Saturated Fat 0.5g • Trans Fat 0.0g • Cholesterol 40mg • Sodium 80mg • Total Carbohydrate 6g • Dietary Fiber 1g • Sugars 1g • Protein 14g

Potato and Spinach Soup

1 Tbsp	olive oil
1	onion, chopped
6 cloves	garlic

❖ In a large pot, heat oil. Cook onions and garlic for 5 minutes.

2 1/2 cups	low-sodium chicken broth
2 1/2 cups	water
1 lb	potatoes, peeled and cubed

❖ Add broth, water, and potatoes; bring to a boil. Reduce heat, and simmer for 20 minutes until potatoes are tender.

1/4 cup	fat-free half and half
2 Tbsp	fat-free sour cream
2 tsp	cayenne pepper
1/4 tsp	pepper
10 oz	spinach, sliced

❖ Gradually stir in half and half, sour cream, cayenne pepper, pepper, and spinach. Simmer for 10 minutes.

Exchanges/Choices
1 Starch • 1 Vegetable • 1/2 Fat

Calories 115 • Calories from Fat 25 • Total Fat 3.0g • Saturated Fat 0.6g • Trans Fat 0.0g • Cholesterol 5mg • Sodium 100mg • Total Carbohydrate 19g • Dietary Fiber 3g • Sugars 3g • Protein 4g

Hot and Spicy Asian Soup

Serves 4 / Serving size: 1/4 recipe

1 cup	low-sodium chicken broth
3 cups	water
2 tsp	low-sodium soy sauce
1 Tbsp	sesame oil
1 cup	sliced scallions
1/2	carrot, thinly sliced, julienned
2 tsp	ground ginger
2 tsp	chili powder

❖ In a large pot, combine all ingredients. Bring to a boil, reduce heat, and simmer for 20 minutes.

Exchanges/Choices

1 Vegetable • 1/2 Fat

Calories 55 • Calories from Fat 35 • Total Fat 4.0g • Saturated Fat 0.6g • Trans Fat 0.0g • Cholesterol 0mg • Sodium 145mg • Total Carbohydrate 4g • Dietary Fiber 1g • Sugars 1g • Protein 2g

Squash Soup

Serves 4 / Serving size: 1/4 recipe

2 cups	low-sodium chicken broth
2 cups	water
1/2 cup	chopped onion
1/2 cup	diced zucchini
1/2 cup	diced yellow squash
1 cup	diced butternut squash
1/4 tsp	dried thyme
1/4 tsp	salt
1/4 tsp	pepper

❖ In a large pot, combine all ingredients. Bring to a boil, reduce heat, and simmer for 20 minutes.

Exchanges/Choices

1 Vegetable

Calories 35 • Calories from Fat 0 • Total Fat 0.0g • Saturated Fat 0.1g • Trans Fat 0.0g • Cholesterol 0mg • Sodium 200mg • Total Carbohydrate 7g • Dietary Fiber 1g • Sugars 2g • Protein 2g

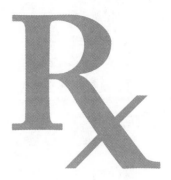

Salads

Spinach Salad

15 oz	fresh baby spinach
1	large tomato, cut into wedges
1 1/2 cups	sliced mushrooms

❖ In a bowl, combine spinach, tomato, and mushrooms.

1	onion, chopped
3 1/2 Tbsp	olive oil
3 Tbsp	red wine vinegar

❖ In a separate bowl, combine onion, oil, and vinegar.

2 Tbsp	bacon bits

❖ Toss vegetables with dressing, and garnish with bacon bits.

Exchanges/Choices
1 Vegetable • 2 Fat

Calories 115 • Calories from Fat 80 • Total Fat 9.0g • Saturated Fat 1.5g • Trans Fat 0.0g • Cholesterol 0mg • Sodium 145mg • Total Carbohydrate 7g • Dietary Fiber 3g • Sugars 2g • Protein 4g

Ambrosia Salad

1	orange, segmented
1	4 oz can pineapple in natural juices, cubed
1	banana, sliced
8	green grapes, halved

❖ Combine fruit, and divide among serving dishes.

1/4 cup	light whipped cream
4 tsp	unsweetened coconut flakes, toasted

❖ Top with a dollop of whipped cream, and garnish with toasted coconut flakes.

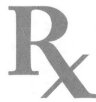

Exchanges/Choices
1/2 Fruit • 1/2 Fat

Calories 55 • Calories from Fat 20 • Total Fat 2.0g • Saturated Fat 1.3g • Trans Fat 0.0g • Cholesterol 5mg • Sodium 0mg • Total Carbohydrate 9g • Dietary Fiber 1g • Sugars 7g • Protein 1g

Coleslaw

1	small head green cabbage, cored and outer leaves removed

❖ Slice the cabbage into thin shreds.

1/4 cup	light mayonnaise
1/4 cup	white vinegar
1 Tbsp	sugar

❖ Combine mayonnaise, vinegar, and sugar; toss mixture with cabbage.

1	carrot, peeled and grated
2 Tbsp	chopped red onion
1 Tbsp	chopped red pepper
1 Tbsp	chopped yellow pepper

❖ Toss in remaining ingredients.

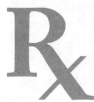

Exchanges/Choices
2 Vegetable • 1/2 Fat

Calories 80 • Calories from Fat 30 • Total Fat 3.5g • Saturated Fat 0.6g • Trans Fat 0.0g • Cholesterol 5mg • Sodium 115mg • Total Carbohydrate 11g • Dietary Fiber 3g • Sugars 7g • Protein 2g

Tabbouleh Salad

4 oz	bulgur wheat

❖ In a small bowl, add bulgur wheat, and cover with cold water. Soak for 20 minutes, and drain well.

2/3 cup	chopped fresh parsley
1/2 cup	diced tomatoes
1 Tbsp	chopped scallions, white parts only

❖ In a large bowl, combine bulgur, parsley, tomatoes, and scallions.

1/4 cup	olive oil
2 Tbsp	lemon juice
1/4 tsp	salt
1/4 tsp	pepper

❖ In a separate bowl, mix oil, lemon juice, salt, and pepper.

❖ Pour over tabbouleh, and toss to coat.

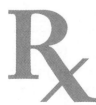

Exchanges/Choices
1/2 Starch • 1 Fat

Calories 95 • Calories from Fat 65 • Total Fat 7.0g • Saturated Fat 1.0g • Trans Fat 0.0g • Cholesterol 0mg • Sodium 80mg • Total Carbohydrate 7g • Dietary Fiber 2g • Sugars 0g • Protein 1g

Potato Salad

1 1/4 lb	potatoes

❖ Preheat oven to 350°F. Place potatoes on a baking pan, and bake for 45 minutes, until tender. Peel and dice potatoes while still hot, and place in a bowl.

6 Tbsp	fat-free mayonnaise
2 oz	red wine vinegar
1 tsp	granulated sugar
1 Tbsp	chopped capers
2 Tbsp	chopped parsley
1/4 tsp	salt
1/2 tsp	pepper

❖ Combine remaining ingredients. Add mixture to potatoes, and toss to coat. Refrigerate salad, and serve cold.

Exchanges/Choices

1 1/2 Starch

Calories 110 • Calories from Fat 10 • Total Fat 1.0g • Saturated Fat 0.2g • Trans Fat 0.0g • Cholesterol 0mg • Sodium 395mg • Total Carbohydrate 24g • Dietary Fiber 2g • Sugars 4g • Protein 2g

Harvest Salad

6 cups	mixed green salad

❖ Wash salad greens, and drain well.

1	yellow tomato, cut into wedges
1	small cucumber, cut into chunks
4	medium thick sliced red onion
1/4 cup	dry roasted walnuts
1/4 cup	dried sweetened cranberries

❖ Toss mixed green salad with other vegetables, walnuts, and cranberries.

4 Tbsp	light raspberry vinaigrette

❖ To avoid wilting, toss mixture with vinaigrette only when ready to serve.

Exchanges/Choices

1/2 Fruit • 1 Vegetable • 1 1/2 Fat

Calories 130 • Calories from Fat 65 • Total Fat 7.0g • Saturated Fat 0.6g • Trans Fat 0.0g • Cholesterol 0mg • Sodium 155mg • Total Carbohydrate 16g • Dietary Fiber 3g • Sugars 10g • Protein 3g

Three-Bean Salad

1	*10.5-oz can no-added-salt chickpeas*
1	*10.5-oz can no-added-salt kidney beans*
1	*14.5-oz can no-added-salt green beans*
2	*large tomatoes, chopped*

❖ Drain canned chickpeas, kidney beans, and green beans, and combine in a large bowl with tomatoes.

1/4 cup	*olive oil*
1/4 cup	*red wine vinegar*
1/2 cup	*chopped shallots*
1 tsp	*salt*
2 tsp	*pepper*

❖ In a separate bowl, combine oil, vinegar, shallots, salt, and pepper. Pour over bean mixture, and toss until well coated.

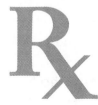

Exchanges/Choices
1/2 Starch • 1 Vegetable • 1 Fat

Calories 120 • Calories from Fat 55 • Total Fat 6.0g • Saturated Fat 0.8g • Trans Fat 0.0g • Cholesterol 0mg • Sodium 240mg • Total Carbohydrate 13g • Dietary Fiber 4g • Sugars 3g • Protein 4g

Pasta Tomato Salad

8 oz	whole-wheat penne pasta

❖ In a large saucepan over medium heat, cook the pasta as directed on the package. Drain and rinse under cold water.

2	medium tomatoes, chopped
1	green onion, with tops, sliced
3 cloves	garlic, minced
1/4 cup	parsley, chopped
1/4 tsp	salt
1/4 tsp	pepper
1 Tbsp	chopped parsley
1/4 cup	olive oil

❖ Mix remaining ingredients, and toss mixture with pasta. Refrigerate, and serve chilled.

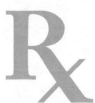

Exchanges/Choices
2 Starch • 2 Fat

Calories 235 • Calories from Fat 90 • Total Fat 10.0g • Saturated Fat 1.3g • Trans Fat 0.0g • Cholesterol 0mg • Sodium 110mg • Total Carbohydrate 32g • Dietary Fiber 5g • Sugars 3g • Protein 5g

Cottage Cheese Tomato Salad

Serves 6 / Serving size: 1/6 recipe

12 oz	*low-fat cottage cheese*
12	*large fresh basil leaves*

❖ Combine cheese and basil, and divide mixture evenly among serving plates.

2 Tbsp	*olive oil*
4 Tbsp	*balsamic vinaigrette*
1	*small red onion, chopped*
1/4 tsp	*salt*
1/4 tsp	*pepper*

❖ Combine oil, vinegar, onion, salt, and pepper.

2	*large tomatoes, seeded and chopped*

❖ Toss dressing with tomatoes. Place tomato mixture on top of cheese mixture.

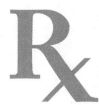

Exchanges/Choices

1 Vegetable • 1 Lean Meat • 1 Fat

Calories 130 • Calories from Fat 70 • Total Fat 8.0g • Saturated Fat 1.3g • Trans Fat 0.0g • Cholesterol 0mg • Sodium 445mg • Total Carbohydrate 7g • Dietary Fiber 1g • Sugars 4g • Protein 8g

Waldorf Salad

4 Tbsp	*nonfat plain yogurt*
1 Tbsp	*fresh lemon juice*
1/4 tsp	*salt*
1/4 tsp	*pepper*

❖ In a large bowl, combine yogurt, lemon juice, salt, and pepper.

2	*sweet apples, cored and chopped*
1/2 cup	*celery, thinly sliced*
1/2 cup	*red seedless grapes, sliced*
1/2 cup	*chopped walnuts, toasted*

❖ Mix apples, celery, grapes, and walnuts; toss with yogurt mixture.

1/2	*head iceberg lettuce*

❖ Slice lettuce into thin shreds. Divide lettuce among serving dishes, and top with fruit mixture.

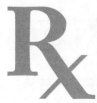

Exchanges/Choices
1 Fruit • 1 Vegetable • 2 Fat

Calories 170 • Calories from Fat 90 • Total Fat 10.0g • Saturated Fat 1.0g • Trans Fat 0.0g • Cholesterol 0mg • Sodium 175mg • Total Carbohydrate 20g • Dietary Fiber 4g • Sugars 14g • Protein 4g

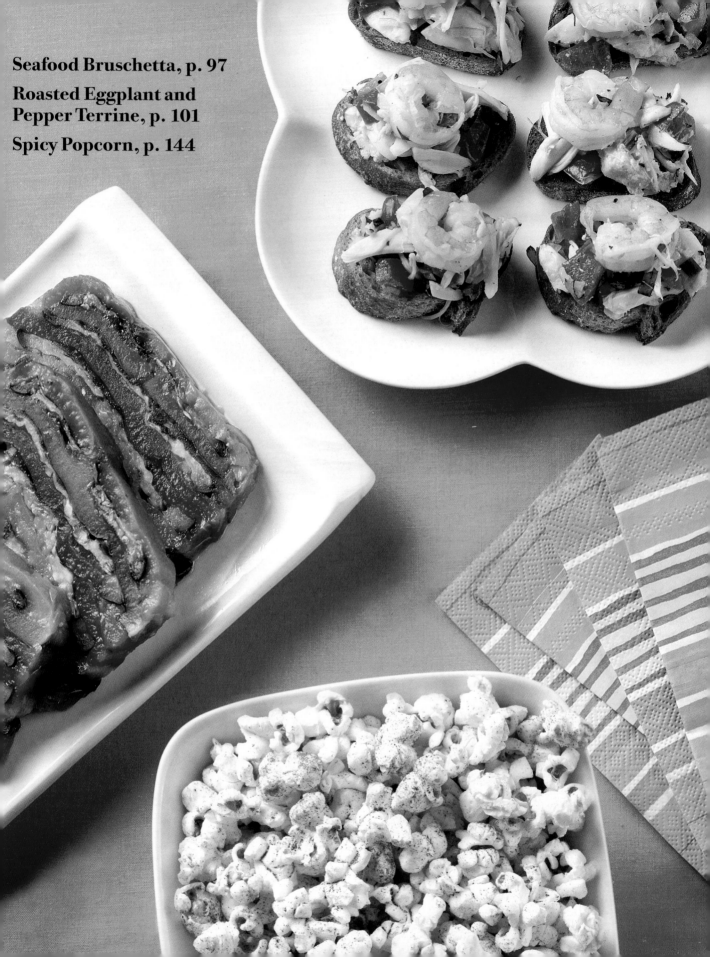

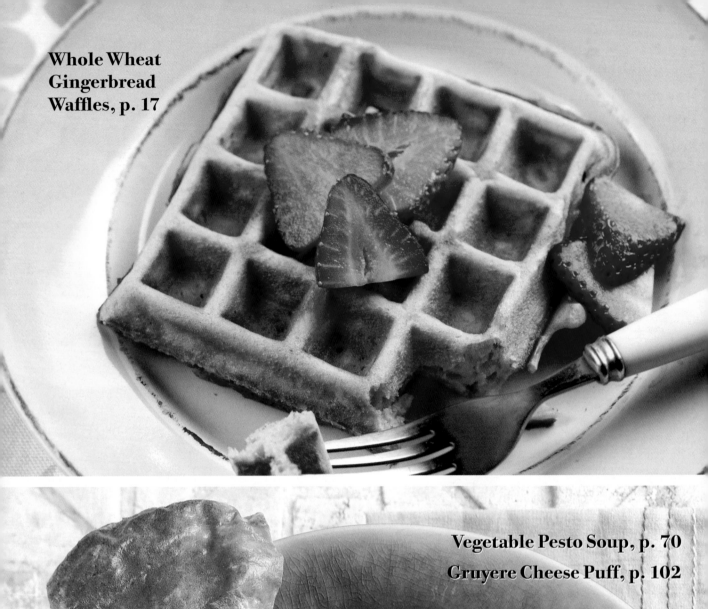

Whole Wheat Gingerbread Waffles, p. 17

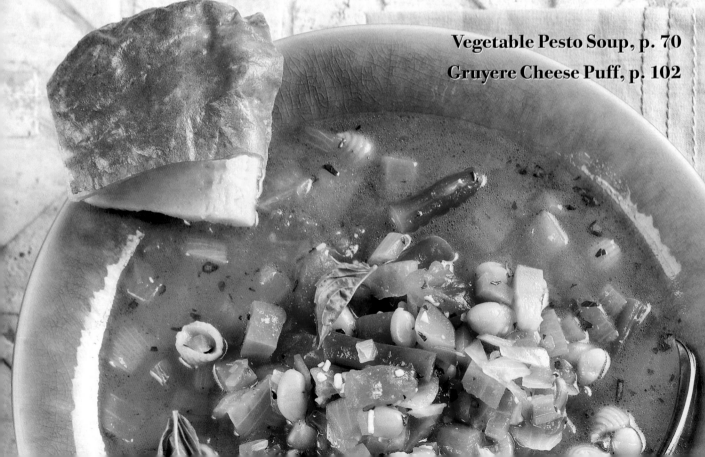

Vegetable Pesto Soup, p. 70

Gruyere Cheese Puff, p. 102

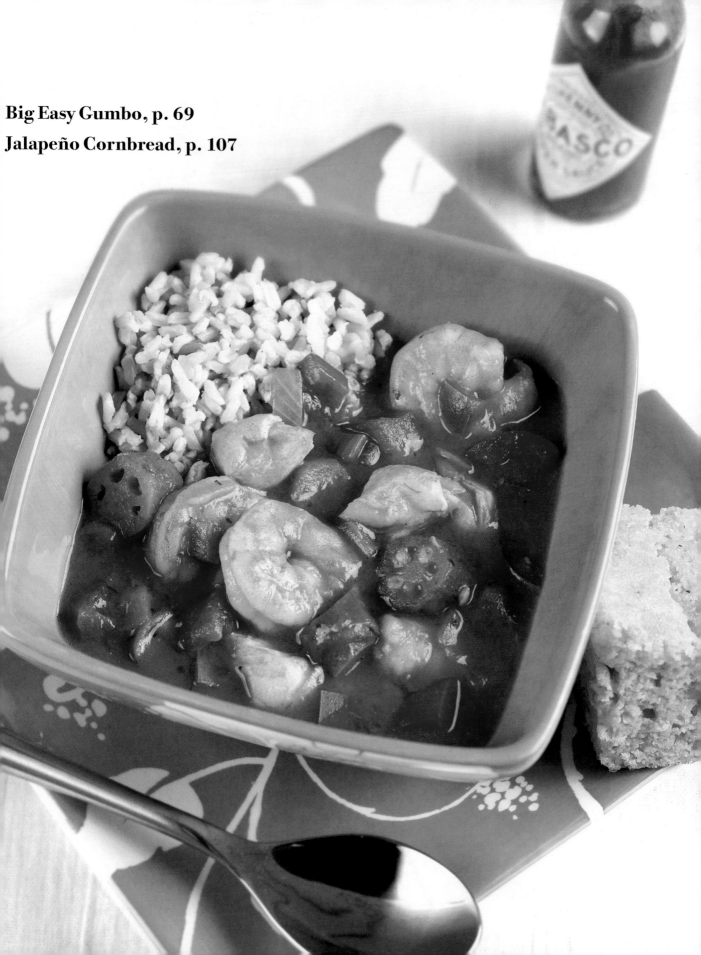

Big Easy Gumbo, p. 69

Jalapeño Cornbread, p. 107

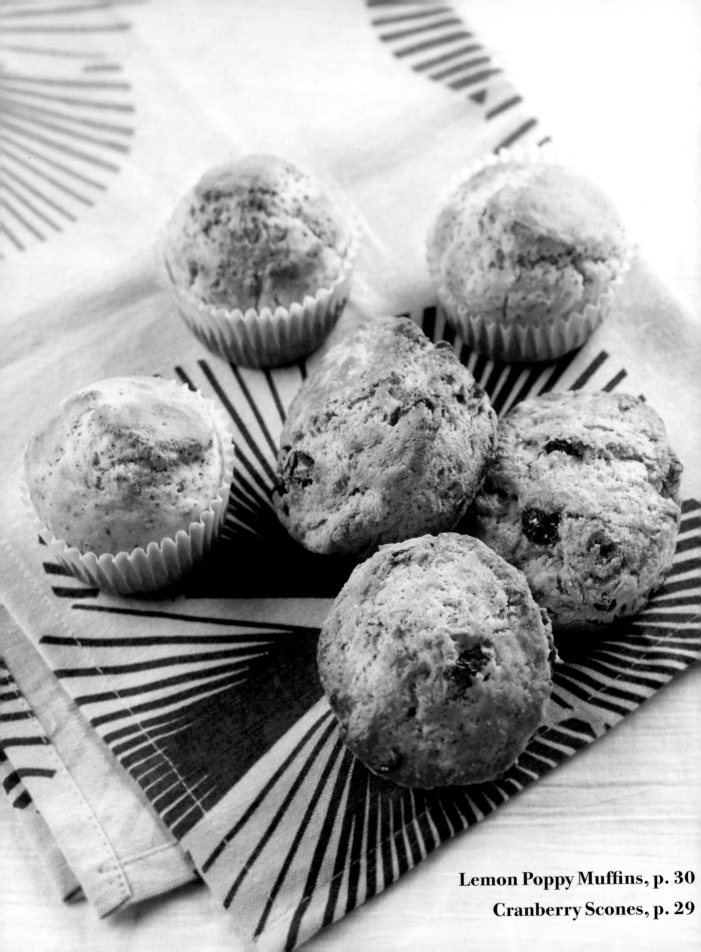

Lemon Poppy Muffins, p. 30
Cranberry Scones, p. 29

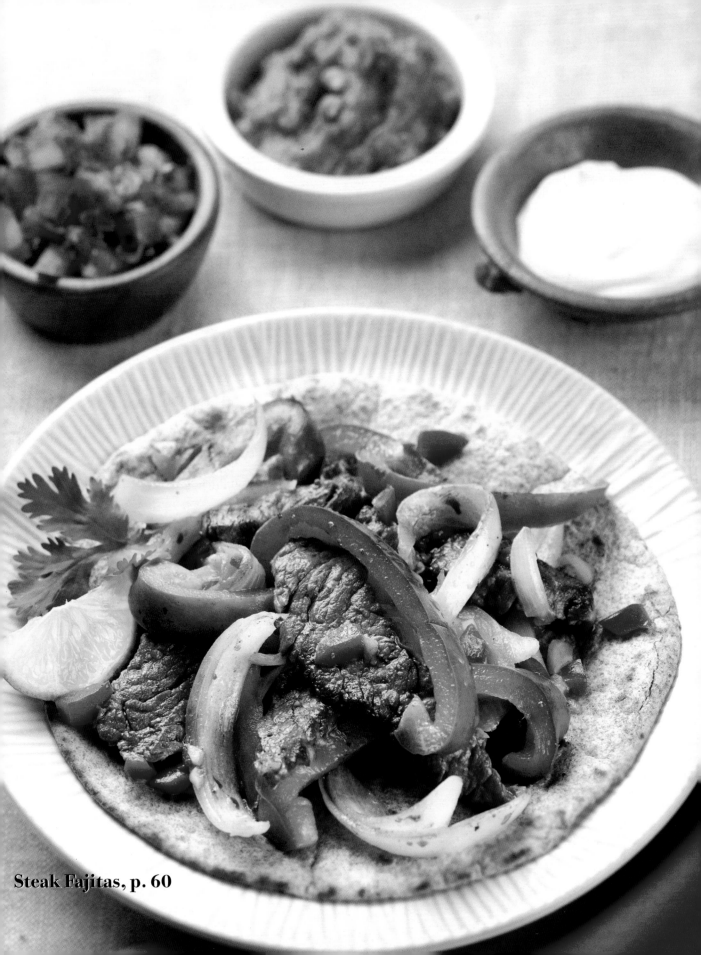

Steak Fajitas, p. 60

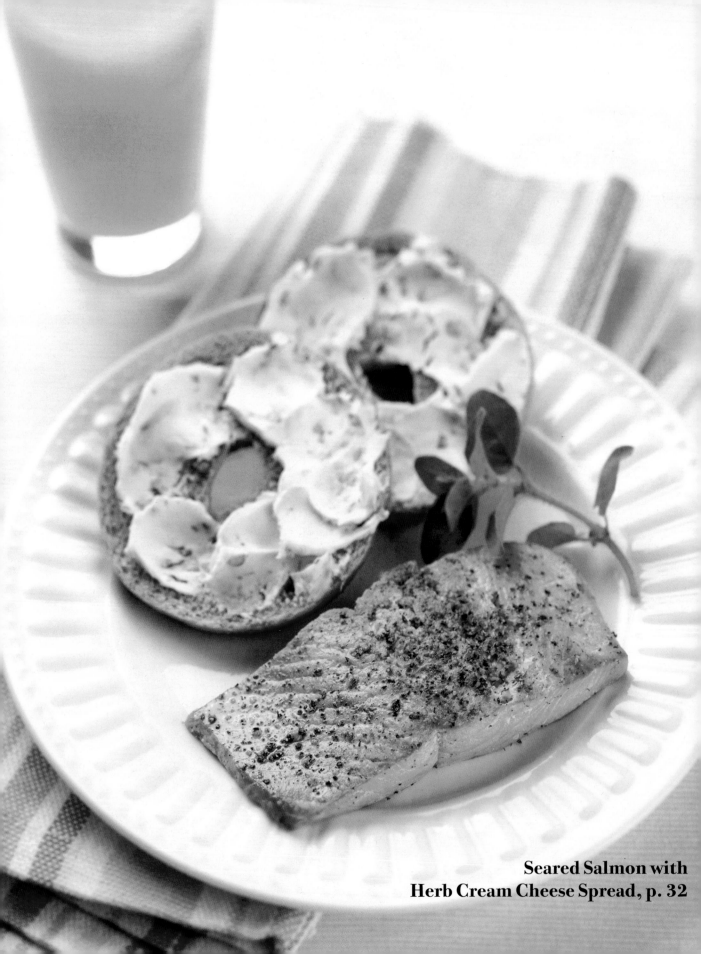

**Seared Salmon with
Herb Cream Cheese Spread, p. 32**

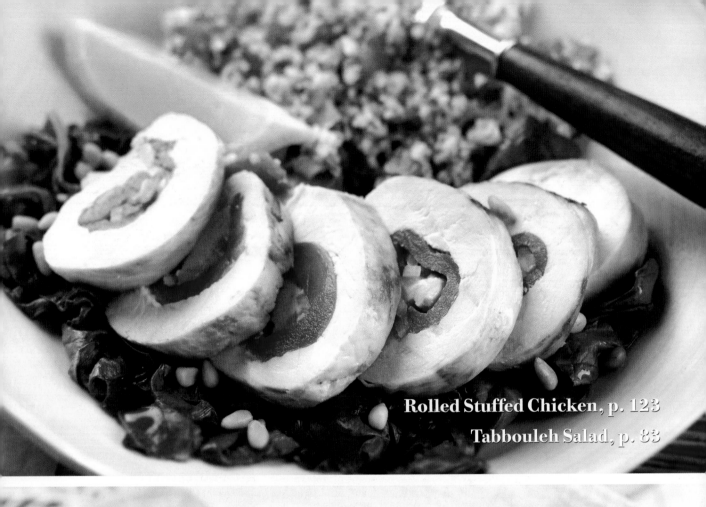

Rolled Stuffed Chicken, p. 123

Tabbouleh Salad, p. 83

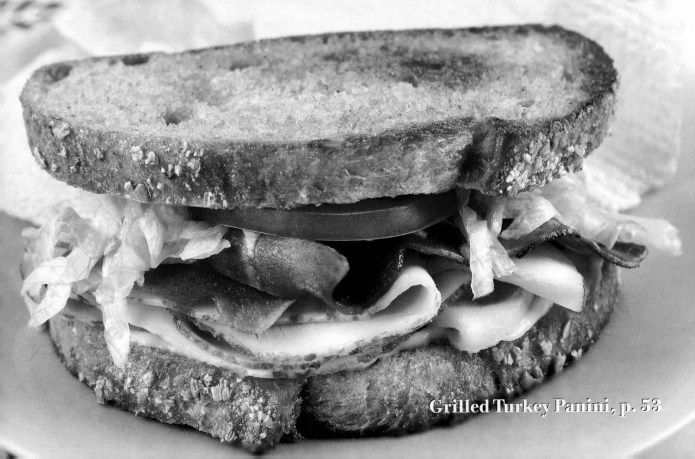

Grilled Turkey Panini, p. 53

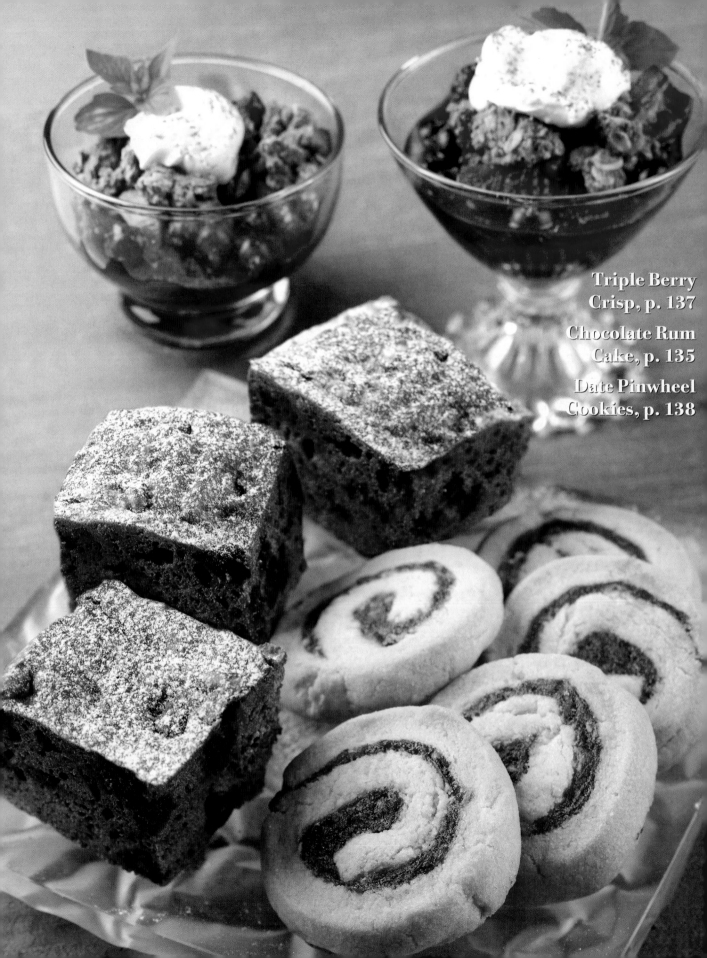

Greek Salad

3 cups	sliced iceberg lettuce
2	large tomatoes, cut into wedges
1/2	cucumber, sliced
1/2	green pepper, sliced
2 oz	reduced-fat feta cheese

❖ In a large bowl, combine lettuce, tomatoes, cucumber, green pepper, and cheese.

2 Tbsp	olive oil
1 Tbsp	lemon juice
3 cloves	garlic
1/2 tsp	dried oregano
1/4 tsp	salt
1/4 tsp	pepper

❖ In a separate bowl, combine oil, lemon juice, garlic, oregano, salt, and pepper. Toss dressing with vegetables.

1	small red onion, sliced
6	kalamata olives

❖ Top with onion and olives.

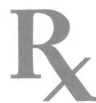

Exchanges/Choices
1 Vegetable • 1 1/2 Fat

Calories 95 • Calories from Fat 55 • Total Fat 6.0g • Saturated Fat 1.5g • Trans Fat 0.0g • Cholesterol 5mg • Sodium 265mg • Total Carbohydrate 8g • Dietary Fiber 2g • Sugars 4g • Protein 3g

Chickpea Salad

1 cup	dried chickpeas
3 cups	water

❖ Rinse chickpeas well with cold water. Soak using the short or long method. Place chickpeas in boiling water, then simmer for 30 minutes or until tender. Drain chickpeas, and rub gently to remove the skins.

1/2 cup	chopped cucumber
1/2 cup	chopped tomatoes

❖ Combine chickpeas, cucumbers, and tomatoes.

1 Tbsp	olive oil
1/4 cup	onions, chopped
6 cloves	garlic, chopped
1 Tbsp	chopped parsley
1/2 tsp	salt
1/2 tsp	pepper
1 Tbsp	lemon juice

❖ Combine oil, onions, garlic, parsley, salt, pepper, and lemon juice. Toss with chickpea mixture.

Prescription for Success

Soak the beans using the short or long method. The short method is to boil the beans for 2 minutes, take the pan off the heat, cover, and let stand for 2 hours. The long method is to soak the chickpeas in water for 8 hours or overnight, placing the pan in the refrigerator. Before cooking them, regardless of method, skim off any skins that float to the surface, drain the soaking liquid, and rinse with clean water.

Exchanges/Choices

2 Starch • 1/2 Vegetable • 1/2 Lean Meat • 1/2 Fat

Calories 210 • Calories from Fat 50 • Total Fat 6.0g • Saturated Fat 0.5g • Trans Fat 0.0g • Cholesterol 0mg • Sodium 310mg • Total Carbohydrate 31g • Dietary Fiber 9g • Sugars 6g • Protein 10g

Belgian Endive and Asparagus Salad

1	bunch asparagus

❖ Cut asparagus on the bias, leaving them long. Take off about one-fourth. Blanch asparagus in boiling water for 1 minute. Immediately place in a bowl of ice water to stop cooking.

2	heads Belgian endive

❖ Wash and dry each leaf of the endive. Julienne endive lengthwise into 4-inch pieces.

1	red pepper, sliced

❖ In a bowl, combine asparagus, endive, and pepper.

1/4 cup	olive oil
1 Tbsp	white wine vinegar
1/4 cup	lemon juice
4 Tbsp	chopped shallots
1/4 tsp	salt
1/2 tsp	pepper

❖ In a small bowl, combine oil, vinegar, lemon juice, shallots, salt, and pepper. Pour mixture over vegetables, and toss to coat well.

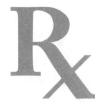

Exchanges/Choices
1 Vegetable • 2 Fat

Calories 115 • Calories from Fat 80 • Total Fat 9.0g • Saturated Fat 1.3g • Trans Fat 0.0g • Cholesterol 0mg • Sodium 120mg • Total Carbohydrate 7g • Dietary Fiber 3g • Sugars 2g • Protein 2g

Beet Salad

Serves 4 / Serving size: 1/4 recipe

| 2 | medium red beets |
| 2 | medium golden beets |

❖ Preheat oven to 350°F.

❖ Leave about 1 inch of the stems and roots attached to the beets. Wrap each beet in foil, and roast in oven for 1 hour. Rub off skins, and cut into wedges.

| 4 Tbsp | balsamic vinegar |
| 1 Tbsp | brown sugar |

❖ In a small saucepan over low heat, add balsamic vinegar and brown sugar. Stir until sugar is dissolved. Continue cooking until liquid has reduced to half, stirring frequently.

| 1/2 tsp | salt |
| 1 1/4 oz | goat cheese |

❖ Spoon reduced balsamic vinegar onto each plate. Divide beets onto each plate, sprinkle with salt, and top with goat cheese.

Prescription for Success
Gently wash beets so the thin skin remains intact. Beets can lose nutrients and color if the skin is broken. Peel beets after they have been cooked.

Exchanges/Choices
1/2 Carbohydrate • 1 Vegetable • 1/2 Fat

Calories 75 • Calories from Fat 20 • Total Fat 2.0g • Saturated Fat 1.3g • Trans Fat 0.0g • Cholesterol 5mg • Sodium 375mg • Total Carbohydrate 12g • Dietary Fiber 1g • Sugars 10g • Protein 3g

Panzanella (Bread Salad)

4 cups	whole-wheat bread, cut into 1/2-inch cubes

❖ Preheat oven to 350°F.

❖ On a large baking pan, spread bread cubes in a single layer. Bake 10 minutes, turning once with a spatula, until golden light brown.

3	large tomatoes, diced
2	cucumbers, peeled, seeded, and diced
1	large red onion, chopped
1/4 cup	green pepper, chopped
1/4 cup	celery, chopped
1/4 cup	chopped fresh basil

❖ Combine the bread with the tomatoes, cucumbers, onion, green pepper, celery, and basil.

1/4 cup	olive oil
2 Tbsp	red wine vinegar
3 cloves	garlic, minced
1/4 tsp	salt
1/4 tsp	pepper

❖ In another bowl, whisk together oil, vinegar, garlic, salt, and pepper. Pour oil mixture over vegetables, and toss to coat.

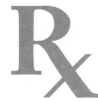

Exchanges/Choices
1/2 Starch • 1 Vegetable • 1 1/2 Fat

Calories 130 • Calories from Fat 65 • Total Fat 7.0g • Saturated Fat 1.1g • Trans Fat 0.1g • Cholesterol 0mg • Sodium 145mg • Total Carbohydrate 13g • Dietary Fiber 3g • Sugars 5g • Protein 3g

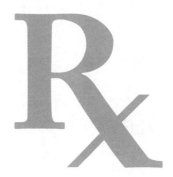

Appetizers

Seafood Bruschetta

8 oz	cooked crabmeat, flaked
4 oz	cooked baby shrimp
2	plum tomatoes, seeded and chopped
1/2 cup	chopped shallots
2 Tbsp	chopped fresh chives
2 Tbsp	chopped fresh basil
1 Tbsp	olive oil
1 Tbsp	lemon juice
4 cloves	garlic, minced
1/2 tsp	pepper

❖ Combine crabmeat, shrimp, tomatoes, shallots, chives, basil, oil, lemon juice, garlic, and pepper. Cover and refrigerate 2 hours to blend flavors.

1/2 lb	baguette, cut into 16 slices
2 Tbsp	olive oil

❖ Preheat oven to 350°F.

❖ Place baguettes slices on a cookie sheet. Brush with oil on both sides, and toast for 8 minutes, turning once. Divide bruschetta evenly among baguette slices.

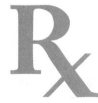

Exchanges/Choices
1/2 Starch • 1 Lean Meat

Calories 90 • Calories from Fat 25 • Total Fat 3.0g • Saturated Fat 0.5g • Trans Fat 0.0g • Cholesterol 30mg • Sodium 150mg • Total Carbohydrate 9g • Dietary Fiber 1g • Sugars 1g • Protein 6g

Mushroom Strudel

	nonstick cooking spray
8 oz	*mushrooms, sliced*
1	*onion, chopped*
4 cloves	*garlic, minced*

❖ Preheat oven to 350°F.

❖ Coat a large sauté pan with cooking spray. Sauté mushrooms, onion, and garlic for 5 minutes.

2 oz	*less-fat cream cheese (Neufchâtel), at room temperature*
1/2 tsp	*salt*
1/2 tsp	*pepper*

❖ Stir in cream cheese, salt, and pepper.

	nonstick cooking spray
6	*14 × 9-inch phyllo sheets, thawed*

❖ Coat a baking sheet with cooking spray. Put one phyllo sheet down on baking sheet, and coat it with cooking spray. Continue until three phyllo sheets are on top of one another.

❖ Top sheets with mushroom mixture, leaving a 1/2-inch space around the edges. Top with three more layers of phyllo, spraying each sheet with cooking spray. Seal edges closed. Bake for 35 minutes, until golden brown. Let cool for 5 minutes before cutting.

Exchanges/Choices
1/2 Starch • 1 Vegetable 1/2 Fat

Calories 80 • Calories from Fat 20 • Total Fat 2.5g • Saturated Fat 1.2g • Trans Fat 0.0g • Cholesterol 5mg • Sodium 285mg • Total Carbohydrate 12g • Dietary Fiber 1g • Sugars 2g • Protein 3g

Crab Dip

8 oz	*fat-free cream cheese*

❖ Place cream cheese in a microwave-safe dish; microwave on high for 30 seconds. Stir until smooth.

8 oz	*cooked crabmeat*
1/4 cup	*green onions, finely chopped*
1 Tbsp	*lemon juice*
1 tsp	*Worcestershire sauce*
1/2 tsp	*paprika*
1 Tbsp	*hot pepper sauce*

❖ Add remaining ingredients. Microwave on high for 1 minute. Serve warm.

Exchanges/Choices
1 Lean Meat

Calories 55 • Calories from Fat 5 • Total Fat 0.5g • Saturated Fat 0.1g • Trans Fat 0.0g • Cholesterol 35mg • Sodium 280mg • Total Carbohydrate 2g • Dietary Fiber 0g • Sugars 1g • Protein 9g

Smoked Salmon Tea Sandwich

6 oz	*fat-free cream cheese*
1/4 cup	*fat-free sour cream*
2 Tbsp	*chopped chives*

❖ Combine cream cheese, sour cream, and chives.

20 slices	*seedless rye bread*

❖ Using a 1 1/2-inch diameter cutter, cut out two circles from each slice of bread.

1 lb	*thinly sliced smoked salmon*

❖ Spread each slice of bread with cheese mixture. Lay salmon slices over half of the bread slices, and top with remaining bread.

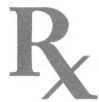

Exchanges/Choices
1/2 Starch • 1 Lean Meat

Calories 75 • Calories from Fat 15 • Total Fat 1.5g • Saturated Fat 0.3g • Trans Fat 0.0g • Cholesterol 5mg • Sodium 325mg • Total Carbohydrate 8g • Dietary Fiber 1g • Sugars 0g • Protein 6g

Tuscan White Bean Spread

Serves 16 / Serving size: 1/16 recipe

2 Tbsp	olive oil
1	onion, chopped
2	shallots, chopped
8 cloves	garlic, chopped

❖ In a small saucepan, combine oil, onion, shallots, and garlic. Cook over medium heat, stirring occasionally, for 3 minutes.

1 Tbsp	red wine vinegar

❖ Add vinegar, and remove from heat.

1	19-oz can white kidney beans, drained and rinsed

❖ In a food processor, purée kidney beans and onion mixture.

1 1/2 tsp	fresh parsley
1 1/2 tsp	fresh basil leaves
1 Tbsp	black pepper
1 Tbsp	lemon juice
1 Tbsp	Worcestershire sauce

❖ Add parsley, basil, pepper, lemon juice, and Worcestershire sauce to food processor and mix until smooth. Transfer to a bowl. Cover and refrigerate. Serve chilled.

Exchanges/Choices
1/2 Starch

Calories 50 • Calories from Fat 20 • Total Fat 2.0g • Saturated Fat 0.3g • Trans Fat 0.0g • Cholesterol 0mg • Sodium 30mg • Total Carbohydrate 7g • Dietary Fiber 2g • Sugars 1g • Protein 2g

Roasted Eggplant and Pepper Terrine

1 tsp	salt
1 lb	peeled eggplant, sliced lengthwise, 1/4 inch thick

❖ Salt eggplant, and let drain on paper towels for 30 minutes.

	nonstick cooking spray
5	red peppers
5	green peppers
4	yellow peppers
4	orange peppers

❖ Spray grill with cooking spray, and place whole peppers on grill. Close the cover, and check on peppers every 2 minutes. Using tongs, turn peppers over so they brown evenly. Place peppers in a closed paper bag or a bowl tightly covered with plastic wrap for 15 minutes. This will allow peppers to steam. Using the back of a knife, scrape off skins. Cut off stems, remove seeds, and cut each pepper into one long piece.

❖ Meanwhile, grill the eggplant.

❖ Line a loaf pan with plastic wrap, leaving an overhang.

1/2 cup	red wine vinegar
3/4 cup	olive oil
1	shallot, minced
1 Tbsp	chopped fresh parsley
1/2 oz	powdered gelatin

❖ In a bowl, combine vinegar, oil, shallot, and parsley. Dissolve the gelatin into the vinaigrette mixture.

❖ In alternating layers, place peppers, eggplant, and vinaigrette mixture until the pan is filled. Cover with overhanging plastic wrap. Weigh down with a 2-lb weight overnight in the refrigerator. Turn terrine onto a plate, and remove plastic wrap. Slice into individual servings.

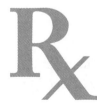

Exchanges/Choices
2 Vegetable • 2 Fat

Calories 145 • Calories from Fat 100 • Total Fat 11.0g • Saturated Fat 1.5g • Trans Fat 0.0g • Cholesterol 0mg • Sodium 150mg • Total Carbohydrate 12g • Dietary Fiber 3g • Sugars 6g • Protein 3g

Gruyere Cheese Puffs

| 1/4 cup | water |
| 2 Tbsp | margarine |

❖ Preheat oven to 350°F.

❖ In a saucepan, combine water and margarine. Bring to a boil.

| 1/4 cup | all-purpose flour |

❖ Add flour. Cook, stirring continuously, until dough comes away from the sides of the pot. Remove from heat.

| 1 | large egg |
| 1/4 cup | gruyere cheese, grated |

❖ Using a hand mixer, mix in egg and cheese. Smooth the mixture onto a parchment-lined baking pan. Bake for 28 minutes, until golden brown. Cut into 24 pieces.

Exchanges/Choices
1/2 Fat

Calories 35 • Calories from Fat 20 • Total Fat 2.5g • Saturated Fat 0.9g • Trans Fat NA • Cholesterol 20mg • Sodium 30mg • Total Carbohydrate 2g • Dietary Fiber 0g • Sugars 0g • Protein 1g

Olive Bread

Serves 16 / Serving size: 1 slice

1/2 Tbsp	*dried yeast*
1/2 tsp	*granulated sugar*
1 oz	*warm water*

❖ Mix yeast and sugar with water. Let the yeast develop for 15 minutes in a warm place.

3 cups	*sifted flour*
1/4 tsp	*salt*
1 1/2 Tbsp	*olive oil*
2 1/2 oz	*warm water*

❖ Add yeast mixture to flour, salt, oil, and water. Knead 8 minutes, until elastic.

2 1/2 oz	*dry-cured olives, pitted and rough chopped*

❖ Add olives; mix well.

1/2 Tbsp	*olive oil*

❖ Rub the oil on the dough, place in a large bowl, and cover with a damp towel. Let rise in a warm place until dough has doubled in volume. When the dough has doubled, knead into loaf shape, cover with a damp towel, and let rise for 1 hour.

❖ Preheat oven to 450°F. Bake for 35 minutes, until the loaf sounds hollow when tapped on the bottom.

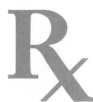

Exchanges/Choices
1 Starch • 1/2 Fat

Calories 110 • Calories from Fat 20 • Total Fat 2.5g • Saturated Fat 0.4g • Trans Fat 0.0g • Cholesterol 0mg • Sodium 180mg • Total Carbohydrate 18g • Dietary Fiber 1g • Sugars 1g • Protein 3g

Marinated Eggplant

Serves 12 / Serving size: 1/12 recipe

3 lb	eggplant
2 tsp	olive oil

❖ Preheat oven to 350°F.

❖ Rub eggplants with olive oil, and bake for 30 minutes. Cut eggplants into 1-inch cubes.

1	small green roasted pepper, chopped
1	small red roasted pepper, chopped

❖ Place eggplants and peppers in a bowl.

1/4 cup	olive oil
1/4 cup	lemon juice
1 tsp	black pepper
6 cloves	garlic, chopped
1 Tbsp	chopped fresh oregano
1 Tbsp	chopped fresh parsley

❖ In another bowl, combine oil, lemon juice, pepper, garlic, oregano, and parsley. Drizzle oil mixture over vegetables. Toss to coat.

Exchanges/Choices
2 Vegetable 1 Fat

Calories 90 • Calories from Fat 55 • Total Fat 6.0g • Saturated Fat 0.8g • Trans Fat 0.0g • Cholesterol 0mg • Sodium 0mg • Total Carbohydrate 11g • Dietary Fiber 3g • Sugars 4g • Protein 1g

Portobello Pâté

1/3 cup	low-sodium chicken broth
1 lb	coarsely chopped portobello mushrooms
1/2 cup	chopped green onions
6 cloves	garlic

❖ In a saucepan, add the broth, mushrooms, onions, and garlic. Bring to a boil, reduce heat, and simmer 10 minutes, until all liquid is absorbed.

4 Tbsp	grated Parmesan cheese
1 Tbsp	balsamic vinegar
1 tsp	lemon juice
1 tsp	Worcestershire sauce
1/2 tsp	salt
1 tsp	pepper

❖ In a blender or food processor, combine mushroom mixture, Parmesan, vinegar, lemon juice, Worcestershire sauce, salt, and pepper. Blend until smooth. Refrigerate for 4 hours to allow flavors to fuse.

32	endive leaves

❖ Spoon the pâté onto endive leaves and serve.

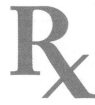

Exchanges/Choices
1 Vegetable

Calories 20 • Calories from Fat 5 • Total Fat 0.5g • Saturated Fat 0.3g • Trans Fat 0.0g • Cholesterol 0mg • Sodium 95mg • Total Carbohydrate 3g • Dietary Fiber 1g • Sugars 1g • Protein 2g

Chicken and Cheese Horns

Serves 20 / Serving size: 1 horn

3 oz	diced gouda cheese
2 cups	diced cooked, skinless, boneless chicken
1	egg yolk
1/4 cup	chopped onion
1/4 cup	chopped fresh parsley
1 tsp	pepper

❖ Combine cheese, chicken, egg yolk, onion, parsley, and pepper.

40	won ton wrappers

❖ Divide filling evenly onto won ton wrappers, and roll into horn shapes.

❖ Preheat oven to 400°F.

❖ Place horns onto parchment-lined baking sheets.

1	large egg, beaten

❖ Brush with beaten egg, and bake 25 minutes, until golden brown.

Exchanges/Choices
1/2 Starch 1 Lean Meat

Calories 80 • Calories from Fat 20 • Total Fat 2.5g • Saturated Fat 1.1g • Trans Fat 0.0g • Cholesterol 40mg • Sodium 120mg • Total Carbohydrate 7g • Dietary Fiber 0g • Sugars 0g • Protein 7g

Jalapeño Cornbread

1 1/2 cups	self-rising cornmeal
1 1/4 cups	2% milk

❖ Preheat oven to 400°F.

❖ In a large bowl, combine cornmeal and milk.

1/4 cup	olive oil
2	large eggs
1 tsp	sugar
1/2 cup	canned creamed corn
2 Tbsp	minced jalapeño peppers
1/4 cup	shredded reduced-fat cheddar cheese
1	small onion, minced

❖ Stir in oil, eggs, sugar, corn, peppers, cheese, and onion.

	nonstick cooking spray

❖ Coat a 12-inch oblong pan with cooking spray. Pour mixture into prepared pan, and bake for 25 minutes, until lightly brown and bread pulls away from the side of the pan.

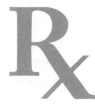

Exchanges/Choices
1 Starch • 1 Fat

Calories 140 • Calories from Fat 55 • Total Fat 6.0g • Saturated Fat 1.4g • Trans Fat 0.0g • Cholesterol 40mg • Sodium 305mg • Total Carbohydrate 18g • Dietary Fiber 1g • Sugars 4g • Protein 4g

Steamed Shrimp
in a Garlic Wine Sauce

Serves 8 / Serving size: 1/8 recipe

2 Tbsp	olive oil
1	large onion, chopped
12 cloves	garlic, coarsely chopped

❖ Heat the oil in a large skillet. Add onion and garlic, and cook for 3 minutes.

2 cups	low-sodium chicken broth
1 1/2 cups	dry white wine
2 lb	shelled, cleaned shrimp

❖ Add broth, wine, and shrimp; cover. Let mixture cook for 5 minutes over medium heat.

1/4 cup	chopped fresh parsley
4	lemons, quartered

❖ Remove from heat, stir in parsley, and serve with lemon wedges.

Exchanges/Choices

1/2 Carbohydrate • 3 Lean Meat

Calories 165 • Calories from Fat 40 • Total Fat 4.5g • Saturated Fat 0.8g • Trans Fat 0.0g • Cholesterol 160mg • Sodium 220mg • Total Carbohydrate 7g • Dietary Fiber 1g • Sugars 2g • Protein 19g

Stuffed Artichokes

6	medium artichokes
1/2	lemon

❖ Wash the artichokes, and dry them upside down, so they can drain. Cut the stems straight across, leaving a level base, so the artichokes will stand upright. Remove the tough outer leaves at the base, and cut about 1/2 inch off the tips of the remaining leaves. Slice 1 inch off the top of the artichokes. As you trim, rub the artichokes with the cut lemon to prevent discoloration.

❖ Preheat oven to 350°F.

2 cups	bread crumbs
6 Tbsp	grated Parmesan cheese
1/2 cup	chopped parsley
6 cloves	garlic, chopped
1/2 tsp	pepper

❖ Combine the bread crumbs, cheese, parsley, garlic, and pepper. Divide the filling among the 6 artichokes, placing some in the center and some between the leaves.

3 Tbsp	olive oil
1 1/2 cups	water

❖ Arrange the artichokes closely together on a baking pan. Pour oil over each, and add water to the bottom of the pan. Cover tightly with foil, and bake for 1 1/2 hours, until the leaves pull out easily.

Exchanges/Choices
2 Starch • 1 Vegetable • 2 Fat

Calories 360 • Calories from Fat 360 • Total Fat 40.0g • Saturated Fat 5.6g • Trans Fat 0.0g • Cholesterol 0mg • Sodium 0mg • Total Carbohydrate 0g • Dietary Fiber 0g • Sugars 0g • Protein 0g

Bean and Avocado Dip

2 cups	cooked pinto beans
1 cup	chopped onion
4 cloves	garlic
1 Tbsp	minced jalapeño pepper
4 Tbsp	chopped cilantro

❖ In a blender or food processor, add beans, onion, garlic, pepper, and cilantro.

1/4 cup	low-sodium chicken broth

❖ Gradually add broth. Blend until smooth.

3	plum tomatoes, peeled, seeded, and chopped
1	avocado, chopped
1 tsp	salt
1 tsp	pepper

❖ In a separate bowl, combine tomatoes, avocado, salt, and pepper.

❖ Add tomato mixture to bean mixture. Refrigerate 4 hours to allow flavors to fuse.

Exchanges/Choices
1/2 Starch • 1 Vegetable

Calories 70 • Calories from Fat 20 • Total Fat 2.0g • Saturated Fat 0.3g • Trans Fat 0.0g • Cholesterol 0mg • Sodium 200mg • Total Carbohydrate 11g • Dietary Fiber 4g • Sugars 1g • Protein 3g

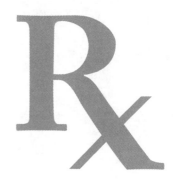

Dinner Entrées

Baked Bass in Fra Diavolo Sauce

1 tsp	olive oil
1	onion, chopped

❖ In a medium saucepan, heat oil. Add onions, and cook for 3 minutes.

1	15-oz can low-sodium tomato sauce
6 cloves	garlic, rough chopped
1 Tbsp	minced jalapeño pepper
1 tsp	sugar

❖ Add tomato sauce, garlic, pepper, and sugar. Cook on low heat for 15 minutes.

1/2 tsp	chopped fresh oregano
1/4 cup	chopped fresh parsley

❖ Remove from heat, and stir in oregano and parsley.

❖ Preheat oven to 350°F.

	nonstick cooking spray
4	bass fillets, about 4 oz each

❖ Coat a baking dish with cooking spray, and place bass fillets in the dish. Top bass with sauce, and bake for 25 minutes, until fish flakes easily when tested with a fork.

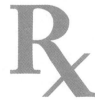

Exchanges/Choices
3 Vegetable (or 1 Carbohydrate) • 2 Lean Meat

Calories 180 • Calories from Fat 30 • Total Fat 3.5g • Saturated Fat 0.8g • Trans Fat 0.0g • Cholesterol 45mg • Sodium 115mg • Total Carbohydrate 15g • Dietary Fiber 4g • Sugars 7g • Protein 23 g

Beef with Oyster Sauce

Serves 4 / Serving size: 1/4 recipe

1 lb	flank steak
2 Tbsp	cornstarch
1	egg white, beaten

❖ Cut beef into three lengthwise strips. Cut strips thinly into 1/8-inch slices. Dredge beef in cornstarch, and coat with egg white.

2 Tbsp	olive oil
2 tsp	minced fresh ginger
3 cloves	garlic, chopped

❖ In a large skillet, heat oil. Add ginger, garlic, and beef, and cook for 3 minutes.

2 Tbsp	oyster sauce
1 Tbsp	soy sauce
2 tsp	sherry
1/2 tsp	sugar
3 oz	canned, sliced water chestnuts
2	green onions, chopped
4	white mushrooms, sliced
2 Tbsp	low-sodium beef broth

❖ Add oyster sauce, soy sauce, sherry, sugar, chestnuts, onions, mushrooms, and broth.

1 tsp	cornstarch
2 tsp	water

❖ Combine cornstarch and water to make a slurry, and slowly stir slurry into beef mixture. Continue stirring until sauce has thickened.

2 cups	cooked white rice

❖ Divide rice on plates, and top with beef with oyster sauce.

Exchanges/Choices
2 Starch • 3 Lean Meat • 2 Fat

Calories 365 • Calories from Fat 115 • Total Fat 13.0g • Saturated Fat 3.5g • Trans Fat 0.0g • Cholesterol 40mg • Sodium 505mg • Total Carbohydrate 33g • Dietary Fiber 2g • Sugars 2g • Protein 27 g

Braised Chicken Breast and Brown Rice

Serves 4 / Serving size: 1/4 recipe

1 Tbsp	olive oil

❖ Preheat oven to 350°F.

❖ In a sauté pan, heat the oil.

1 lb	boneless, skinless chicken breasts
1/2 tsp	salt
1 tsp	pepper

❖ Season the chicken with salt and pepper. Add chicken to sauté pan, and cook for 2 minutes on each side. Transfer chicken to a baking dish, and set aside.

1	onion, chopped

❖ Add onions to sauté pan, and cook for 3 minutes.

4 cloves	garlic, chopped
1 stalk	sliced celery
1	carrot, peeled and sliced
1	sprig fresh rosemary
3 1/2 cups	water
1 cup	uncooked brown rice

❖ Add garlic, celery, carrot, rosemary, water, rice, and chicken to baking dish. Bake for 40 minutes, until chicken is fully cooked.

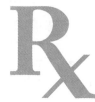

Exchanges/Choices
2 1/2 Starch • 1 Vegetable • 3 Lean Meat

Calories 360 • Calories from Fat 70 • Total Fat 8.0g • Saturated Fat 1.6g • Trans Fat 0.0g • Cholesterol 65mg • Sodium 385mg • Total Carbohydrate 42g • Dietary Fiber 3g • Sugars 3g • Protein 29 g

Roasted Turkey Breast with Vegetables

Serves 6 / Serving size: 1/6 recipe

1 1/2 lb	boneless, skinless turkey breast
1 tsp	olive oil
1 tsp	paprika

❖ Preheat oven to 350°F.

❖ Place turkey breast on rack in roasting pan. Brush turkey breast with olive oil. Sprinkle with paprika.

1/2 cup	chopped onion
1/2 cup	low-sodium chicken broth
1 cup	water

❖ To the bottom of roasting pan, add onion, broth, and enough water to just reach the bottom of the turkey breast.

6	turnips, peeled
6	carrots, peeled
2 tsp	olive oil
1 tsp	pepper

❖ Slice turnips 3/4 of the way through, and cut carrots into 2-inch pieces. Brush vegetables with oil, and sprinkle with pepper. Place vegetables along the side of the turkey breast.

❖ Cover and roast in preheated oven for 40 minutes until fully cooked. Remove turkey and keep warm.

❖ Strain drippings into a pan, and skim off any excess fat. Heat the drippings to a boil.

2 tsp	cornstarch
4 tsp	water

❖ Combine cornstarch and water to make a slurry. Slowly stir in the slurry, and cook for 2 minutes, until thickened.

❖ Slice turkey, and serve with gravy and vegetables.

Exchanges/Choices

3 Vegetable • 3 Lean Meat

Calories 205 • Calories from Fat 25 • Total Fat 3.0g • Saturated Fat 0.6g • Trans Fat 0.0g • Cholesterol 75mg • Sodium 115mg • Total Carbohydrate 14g • Dietary Fiber 4g • Sugars 7g • Protein 29 g

Vegetable Lasagna

1/2 cup	sliced onion
6 cloves	garlic, chopped
3	tomatoes, peeled and sliced
1/2 lb	eggplant, peeled and sliced lengthwise
1	small zucchini, sliced lengthwise
1/2 cup	sliced mushrooms
1 tsp	dried oregano
1 tsp	black pepper
1 Tbsp	olive oil

❖ Preheat oven to 375°F.

❖ In a large baking pan, combine onion, garlic, tomatoes, eggplant, zucchini, mushrooms, oregano, and black pepper. Coat with oil, and roast in preheated oven for 10 minutes.

2	eggs, beaten
1 cup	part-skim ricotta cheese
1/4 cup	chopped fresh parsley

❖ In a bowl, combine eggs, ricotta cheese, and parsley; set aside.

	nonstick cooking spray
1/2 lb	lasagna noodles, cooked
1 Tbsp	freshly grated Parmesan cheese

❖ Coat a baking dish with cooking spray. To assemble lasagna, first layer pan with noodles, top with a portion of vegetables, and then top with ricotta mixture. Repeat layers, ending with pasta. Cover and bake for 20 minutes. Sprinkle with remaining Parmesan, cover, and bake 5 minutes.

Exchanges/Choices
2 Starch • 2 Vegetable • 1 Lean Meat • 1 Fat

Calories 280 • Calories from Fat 70 • Total Fat 8.0g • Saturated Fat 3.2g • Trans Fat 0.0g • Cholesterol 85mg • Sodium 90mg • Total Carbohydrate 39g • Dietary Fiber 4g • Sugars 6g • Protein 14 g

Roast Beef

Serves 6 / Serving size: 1/6 recipe

1 1/2 lb	boneless beef eye round roast, trimmed of excess fat
1/4 tsp	salt
1 Tbsp	cracked black pepper

❖ Preheat oven to 400°F.

❖ Season the beef with salt and pepper. Place beef on rack in roasting pan.

3 cloves	garlic
1/2 cup	chopped onion
1 cup	water

❖ To the bottom of roasting pan, add garlic, onion, and enough water to just reach the bottom of the beef. Roast uncovered for 75 minutes until desired doneness is reached.

Exchanges/Choices
4 Lean Meat

Calories 155 • Calories from Fat 30 • Total Fat 3.5g • Saturated Fat 1.3g • Trans Fat 0.0g • Cholesterol 50mg • Sodium 135mg • Total Carbohydrate 3g • Dietary Fiber 1g • Sugars 1g • Protein 27 g

Turkey Vegetable Loaf

Serves 4 / Serving size: 1/4 recipe

	nonstick cooking spray

❖ Preheat oven to 350°F. Coat a loaf pan with cooking spray.

3/4 lb	ground turkey
1/2 cup	egg substitute
1/2 cup	oatmeal
1/2 cup	peeled carrots
1/4 cup	chopped onion
1/4 cup	chopped fresh parsley
1/2 tsp	salt

❖ In a large bowl, combine all ingredients. Using your hands, mix ingredients well. Place mixture into the loaf pan. Bake loaf for 40 minutes.

Exchanges/Choices
1/2 Starch • 3 Lean Meat • 1 Fat

Calories 210 • Calories from Fat 90 • Total Fat 10.0g • Saturated Fat 2.8g • Trans Fat 0.2g • Cholesterol 65mg • Sodium 470mg • Total Carbohydrate 10g • Dietary Fiber 2g • Sugars 2g • Protein 20 g

Chicken and Bulgur Wheat Cups

Serves 6 / Serving size: 1/6 recipe

	nonstick cooking spray
1 lb	ground chicken breast
1 stalk	celery, chopped
1	small onion, chopped

❖ Coat a sauté pan with cooking spray, and heat the pan over medium-high heat. Add chicken, celery, and onion, and cook for 5 minutes, stirring frequently.

1/2 cup	uncooked cracked bulgur wheat
1/2 cup	water
1 cup	low-sodium chicken broth
1 tsp	pepper
1 Tbsp	chopped fresh dill weed
1/2 cup	sliced white mushrooms

❖ Stir in bulgur, water, broth, pepper, dill, and mushrooms. Bring to a boil, reduce heat, and cover. Simmer for 25 minutes, until wheat is tender and liquid is absorbed.

2	whole eggs, lightly beaten
3 oz	shredded reduced-fat cheddar cheese

❖ Let mixture cool slightly. Stir in eggs and cheese.

❖ Preheat oven to 350°F.

	nonstick cooking spray
12	9 × 14-inch frozen phyllo sheets

❖ Coat six 12-oz ramekin baking dishes with cooking spray. Lightly spray each phyllo sheet with cooking spray to prevent them from drying out. Place phyllo sheets in the ramekin dish, overlapping the sides. Evenly distribute chicken mixture among ramekins, and fold overlapping phyllo to cover mixture. Place dishes on baking sheet, and bake for 45 minutes, until golden brown.

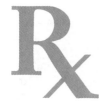

Exchanges/Choices
1 1/2 Starch • 3 Lean Meat

Calories 265 • Calories from Fat 55 • Total Fat 6.0g • Saturated Fat 1.9g • Trans Fat 0.0g • Cholesterol 125mg • Sodium 285mg • Total Carbohydrate 24g • Dietary Fiber 3g • Sugars 1g • Protein 28 g

Roasted Pork Teriyaki with Potatoes and Sweet Apple Topping

Serves 6 / Serving size: 1/6 recipe

1/4 cup	teriyaki sauce
2 tsp	Worcestershire sauce
3 cloves	garlic, chopped

❖ Combine teriyaki sauce, Worcestershire sauce, and garlic.

1 1/2 lb	trimmed, boneless pork loin

❖ Marinate pork in teriyaki mixture for at least 1 hour in the refrigerator.

❖ Preheat oven to 350°F. Place pork in a roasting pan.

1/4 cup	water

❖ Pour marinade over pork, and add water to bottom of pan. Roast pork uncovered in the preheated oven for 1 hour, 15 minutes, until done.

3	potatoes, cubed (about 1 1/2 lb total)
1 tsp	olive oil
1/2 tsp	oregano
1/2 tsp	thyme

❖ Coat the potatoes with oil, and season with oregano and thyme. Bake in 350°F oven for 40 minutes, until brown.

1 1/2 cups	peeled, chopped McIntosh apples
1/4 cup	golden raisins
1 Tbsp	brown sugar
1/4 tsp	ground nutmeg
1/4 tsp	ground cinnamon

❖ Meanwhile, combine apples, raisins, brown sugar, nutmeg, and cinnamon in a small pan. Cook mixture over medium heat, stirring frequently, for 7 minutes, until apples have softened. Portion roast onto plates, top with apple mixture, and serve with potatoes.

Exchanges/Choices
1 Starch • 1 Fruit • 3 Lean Meat • 1/2 Fat

Calories 290 • Calories from Fat 70 • Total Fat 8.0g • Saturated Fat 3.0g • Trans Fat 0.0g • Cholesterol 50mg • Sodium 515mg • Total Carbohydrate 31g • Dietary Fiber 3g • Sugars 12g • Protein 23 g

Lobster in Cumin Sauce

Serves 4 / Serving size: 1/4 recipe

1 cup	low-sodium chicken broth
1/4 cup	water
1 Tbsp	ground cumin
1/2 cup	chopped shallots
6 cloves	garlic

❖ Add broth, water, cumin, shallots, and garlic to a saucepan. Bring to a boil.

1 lb	lobster meat

❖ Lower heat to medium, and add lobster. Cook for 5 minutes, until meat is opaque.

2 Tbsp	fresh chopped cilantro

❖ Stir in chopped cilantro.

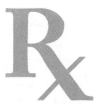

Exchanges/Choices

1 Vegetable • 2 Lean Meat

Calories 120 • Calories from Fat 10 • Total Fat 1.0g • Saturated Fat 0.2g • Trans Fat 0.0g • Cholesterol 65mg • Sodium 380mg • Total Carbohydrate 7g • Dietary Fiber 1g • Sugars 1g • Protein 21 g

Honey Lemon Chicken

Serves 4 / Serving size: 1/4 recipe

2 Tbsp	honey
2 Tbsp	freshly squeezed lemon juice
4 cloves	garlic, minced
1/2 tsp	black pepper

❖ Preheat oven to 375°F.

❖ In a bowl, combine honey, lemon juice, garlic, and pepper.

8	boneless, skinless chicken thighs

❖ Coat chicken with honey mixture, and arrange in a baking dish. Bake for 40 minutes, until juices run clear when chicken is pierced.

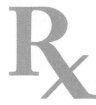

Exchanges/Choices

1/2 Carbohydrate • 4 Lean Meat • 1 Fat

Calories 255 • Calories from Fat 100 • Total Fat 11.0g • Saturated Fat 3.2g • Trans Fat 0.0g • Cholesterol 100mg • Sodium 95mg • Total Carbohydrate 10g • Dietary Fiber 0g • Sugars 9g • Protein 27 g

Chicken Marsala

Serves 4 / Serving size: 1/4 recipe

2 Tbsp	olive oil

❖ In a skillet, heat the oil.

1 lb	boneless, skinless chicken breasts
4 Tbsp	all-purpose flour
2	egg whites, beaten

❖ Dredge chicken in flour; then dip in egg whites.

❖ Cook chicken in oil until golden brown.

1 Tbsp	all-purpose flour
1 Tbsp	margarine

❖ In a separate pan, combine flour and margarine to prepare a roux. Cook for 10 minutes over low heat.

❖ Transfer chicken from skillet to a baking dish.

2 cups	sliced white mushrooms
1 cup	small onion wedges
3 cloves	garlic, chopped

❖ Add mushrooms, onion, and garlic to skillet. Sauté for 3 minutes.

1 tsp	black pepper
1/2 cup	low-sodium chicken broth
1/4 cup	marsala cooking wine

❖ Add mushroom mixture to roux. Stir in pepper, broth, and wine. Simmer for 15 minutes, stirring frequently.

❖ Preheat oven to 350°F. Top chicken with marsala sauce. Bake for 45 minutes.

4 Tbsp	fat-free sour cream

❖ Top each serving with 1 Tbsp sour cream.

Exchanges/Choices
1/2 Starch • 1 Vegetable • 4 Lean Meat • 1 Fat

Calories 295 • Calories from Fat 110 • Total Fat 12.0g • Saturated Fat 2.4g • Trans Fat 0.0g • Cholesterol 70mg • Sodium 140mg • Total Carbohydrate 16g • Dietary Fiber 1g • Sugars 3g • Protein 29 g

Rolled Stuffed Chicken

Serves 4 / Serving size: 1/4 recipe

1 lb	boneless, skinless chicken breasts

❖ Place each chicken breast between two pieces of plastic wrap. Lightly pound chicken to 1/4 inch thickness. Discard plastic when done.

1	large roasted red pepper, sliced julienne
1/4 cup	chopped shallots

❖ Combine red pepper and shallots, and top each chicken breast with mixture.

❖ Starting from one end, roll up chicken. Secure with wooden toothpicks.

❖ Preheat oven to 350°F.

1 Tbsp	olive oil

❖ Brush each chicken roll with oil, and place in a baking dish. Bake for 40 minutes, until chicken is no longer pink.

1/4 cup	low-sodium chicken broth
10 oz	fresh spinach
4 tsp	bacon bits

❖ In a saucepan, combine broth, spinach, and bacon bits. Cook for 5 minutes, until spinach has wilted.

2 Tbsp	pine nuts, lightly toasted

❖ Divide spinach evenly among plates, top with sliced chicken rolls, and garnish with pine nuts.

℞ Prescription for Success

The easy way to roast a pepper:
- Wash and dry the pepper.
- Coat pepper in 1 tsp olive oil, and roast in a shallow dish for 30 minutes until tender.
- Another method is to directly place the pepper on a gas burner (no oil needed), turning occasionally until evenly blackened.

After roasting, place the pepper in a brown paper bag, and let rest for 15 minutes. Using a knife, scrape off the skin. Slice the pepper, and discard stem and seeds.

Exchanges/Choices

1 Vegetable • 4 Lean Meat • 1 Fat

Calories 235 • Calories from Fat 90 • Total Fat 10.0g • Saturated Fat 1.9g • Trans Fat 0.0g • Cholesterol 70mg • Sodium 205mg • Total Carbohydrate 8g • Dietary Fiber 3g • Sugars 3g • Protein 29 g

Meatballs with Fettuccini and Red Sauce

1 lb	ground chicken breast
3	whole eggs
2	egg whites
1 cup	plain dried bread crumbs
1 tsp	garlic powder
1 tsp	black pepper

❖ In a large bowl, combine chicken, eggs, egg whites, bread crumbs, garlic powder, and black pepper. Roll mixture into 12 meatballs.

❖ Preheat oven to 350°F.

	nonstick cooking spray

❖ Coat a baking pan with cooking spray. Place meatballs on pan, and cook for 30 minutes, turning occasionally.

1	14 1/2 oz can low-sodium diced tomatoes
1/4 cup	chopped onion
3 cloves	garlic, chopped
1 tsp	dried basil
1/2 tsp	dried oregano
1 tsp	sugar

❖ In a large saucepan, combine tomatoes, onion, garlic, basil, oregano, and sugar. Cook over low heat, stirring occasionally.

3/4 lb	spinach fettuccine, cooked

❖ Mix fettuccine with sauce, and divide evenly among plates. Top dishes with two meatballs each.

Exchanges/Choices
2 Starch • 1 Vegetable • 3 Lean Meat

Calories 310 • Calories from Fat 55 • Total Fat 6.0g • Saturated Fat 1.7g • Trans Fat 0.0g • Cholesterol 155mg • Sodium 235mg • Total Carbohydrate 34g • Dietary Fiber 3g • Sugars 4g • Protein 29 g

Pineapple Pepper Steak

1 lb	lean flank steak

❖ Cut beef into three lengthwise strips. Cut strips thinly into 1/8-inch slices.

2 Tbsp	cornstarch
1	egg white, beaten

❖ Dredge beef in cornstarch, and coat with egg white.

2 Tbsp	olive oil

❖ In a large skillet, heat the oil. Cook beef for 3 minutes, stirring occasionally.

2 cups	fresh pineapple, cut into chunks
1	red pepper, sliced
1	green pepper, sliced
1 Tbsp	minced jalapeño pepper
1	carrot, sliced
1	scallion, sliced
8 cloves	garlic, chopped

❖ In a bowl, combine pineapple, peppers, carrot, scallion, and garlic. Add mixture to beef.

1 tsp	cornstarch
2 tsp	water

❖ Combine cornstarch and water to make a slurry. Slowly add slurry to pan, and continue stirring until sauce has thickened.

3 cups	cooked brown rice

❖ Divide rice evenly among plates, and top with pineapple pepper steak.

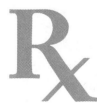

Exchanges/Choices

1 1/2 Starch • 1/2 Fruit • 1 Vegetable • 2 Lean Meat • 1 Fat

Calories 310 • Calories from Fat 90 • Total Fat 10.0g • Saturated Fat 2.5g • Trans Fat 0.0g • Cholesterol 25mg • Sodium 55mg • Total Carbohydrate 37g • Dietary Fiber 4g • Sugars 8g • Protein 19 g

Grilled Chicken over Whole-Wheat Pasta and Vegetables

1 lb	boneless, skinless chicken breast

❖ Place each chicken breast between two pieces of plastic wrap. Lightly pound chicken to 1/4 inch thickness. Discard plastic when done.

1 tsp	pepper

❖ Season the chicken with pepper.

	nonstick cooking spray

❖ Coat a grill with cooking spray, and heat on medium. Cook chicken on hot grill for 10 minutes, turning over for even cooking. Cut cooked chicken into bite-sized chunks.

1/2 lb	whole-wheat spaghetti

❖ Cook spaghetti in 2 1/2 quarts of boiling water for 6 minutes until al dente; drain well.

3 Tbsp	olive oil
1	small onion, minced
1	medium roasted red pepper, sliced
8 cloves	garlic

❖ In a sauté pan over high heat, cook olive oil, onion, red pepper, and whole garlic cloves for 2 minutes.

1/2 cup	low-sodium chicken broth
10 oz	fresh spinach

❖ To pan, add chicken broth, chicken, and spinach; cook 5 minutes, until spinach has wilted. Remove from heat, and toss with pasta.

Exchanges/Choices
2 1/2 Starch • 2 Vegetable • 4 Lean Meat • 1 Fat

Calories 475 • Calories from Fat 125 • Total Fat 14.0g • Saturated Fat 2.4g • Trans Fat 0.0g • Cholesterol 65mg • Sodium 130mg • Total Carbohydrate 50g • Dietary Fiber 9g • Sugars 4g • Protein 36 g

Asian Thighs

1 Tbsp	hoisin sauce
1/3 cup	molasses
4 Tbsp	lime juice
2 Tbsp	reduced-sodium soy sauce
2 Tbsp	grated fresh ginger
1 Tbsp	sesame oil
1 Tbsp	dried red pepper
1 tsp	black pepper
1 tsp	garlic powder

❖ Combine ingredients in a bowl; mix well.

8	boneless, skinless chicken thighs

❖ Dip chicken in marinade to cover all sides. Arrange chicken in a shallow pan; pour remaining marinade over chicken. Cover and refrigerate for 3 hours or overnight.

❖ Broil chicken for 6 minutes on each side, until fully cooked.

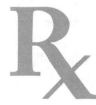

Exchanges/Choices
1 1/2 Carbohydrate • 4 Lean Meat • 1 1/2 Fat

Calories 350 • Calories from Fat 135 • Total Fat 15.0g • Saturated Fat 3.7g • Trans Fat 0.0g • Cholesterol 100mg • Sodium 445mg • Total Carbohydrate 25g • Dietary Fiber 1g • Sugars 18g • Protein 28 g

Spinach and Rice Stuffed Pork with Fruit Wine Sauce

Serves 4 / Serving size: 1/4 recipe

4	*1 1/2-inch thick lean boneless pork chops, about 5 oz each*
1 tsp	*pepper*

❖ Cut a deep pocket in the side of the chops. Trim off excess fat, and season with pepper.

1/4 cup	*minced onion*
2 tsp	*olive oil*
1/2 cup	*raw long-grain rice*

❖ In a large pan, sauté onion in oil. Stir in rice, and cook 2 minutes, until lightly browned.

1 1/2 cups	*low-sodium chicken broth*
3 cloves	*garlic, chopped*
4 Tbsp	*chopped fresh basil*

❖ Add chicken broth, garlic, and basil. Reduce heat, cover, and do not stir. Cook 20 minutes.

10 oz	*fresh spinach*

❖ Stir in spinach. Continue cooking until liquid is absorbed. Fluff rice with a fork.

❖ Preheat oven to 350°F. Stuff pork chops with rice mixture. Extra stuffing may be divided onto plates when serving.

1 tsp	*olive oil*

❖ Over high heat, add olive oil to a large ovenproof sauté pan. Add pork chops, and brown on each side. Place pan in preheated oven, and cook for 40 minutes, turning once.

3/4 cup	*port wine*
1/4 cup	*balsamic vinegar*
1 cup	*blackberries*
1 cup	*raspberries*

❖ To another pan, over medium heat, add wine, vinegar, and berries. Cook until liquid reduces by half.

1	*Bosc pear, peeled, cored, cut into 12 slices*

❖ Coat pear slices with wine mixture. Divide any extra rice evenly among plates. Top rice with pork chops, sliced pear, and fruit wine sauce.

Exchanges/Choices
1 Starch • 1 Fruit • 1 Vegetable • 4 Lean Meat • 1 1/2 Fat

Calories 445 • Calories from Fat 115 • Total Fat 13.0g • Saturated Fat 4.2g • Trans Fat 0.0g • Cholesterol 65mg • Sodium 135mg • Total Carbohydrate 43g • Dietary Fiber 7g • Sugars 12g • Protein 31 g

Seared Steak Tidbits

2	medium potatoes

❖ Wash potatoes. Fill a pot with enough water to cover potatoes, and cook 20 minutes, until tender.

1 1/2 tsp	seasoned meat tenderizer
2 Tbsp	black pepper
3/4 lb	lean steak, cubed

❖ Sprinkle tenderizer and pepper on steak, covering all sides.

	nonstick cooking spray

❖ Spray a large sauté pan with nonstick cooking spray, and heat over high heat. Cook steak cubes for 8 minutes, turning frequently to brown all sides.

1 tsp	paprika

❖ Cut potatoes into cubes, and sprinkle with paprika. Serve with steak tidbits.

Prescription for Success
Serve with Harvest Salad (p. 84).

Exchanges/Choices
1 1/2 Starch • 2 Lean Meat

Calories 200 • Calories from Fat 40 • Total Fat 4.5g • Saturated Fat 1.5g • Trans Fat 0.1g • Cholesterol 55mg • Sodium 480mg • Total Carbohydrate 20g • Dietary Fiber 3g • Sugars 1g • Protein 21 g

Seared Chicken and Butternut Squash

Serves 8 / Serving size: 1/8 recipe

2 1/2 lb	boneless, skinless chicken breasts

❖ Slice chicken into eight equal portions.

1 Tbsp	olive oil

❖ In a large saucepan, heat oil over medium-high heat. Sear chicken, turning once, until brown on both sides. Transfer chicken to a plate.

4 cups	butternut squash, peeled and cut into small cubes
1	medium onion, chopped
8 cloves	garlic, chopped
1 tsp	dried rosemary
1 tsp	dried thyme
1 Tbsp	black pepper

❖ To the same saucepan, add butternut squash, onion, garlic, rosemary, thyme, and pepper; stir often for 5 minutes.

1 cup	low-sodium chicken broth
4	bay leaves
2 cups	diced plum tomatoes
1 Tbsp	minced jalapeño pepper
1/4 cup	orange juice
2 Tbsp	Worcestershire sauce

❖ Add broth, bay leaves, tomatoes, jalapeño pepper, orange juice, and Worcestershire sauce. Return chicken and accumulated juices to pan. Cover, reduce heat, and simmer for 25 minutes, until chicken is fully cooked and squash is tender.

20 oz	fresh baby spinach

❖ Stir in spinach, and cook for 4 minutes until wilted.

Exchanges/Choices
1/2 Starch • 2 Vegetable • 4 Lean Meat

Calories 250 • Calories from Fat 55 • Total Fat 6.0g • Saturated Fat 1.4g • Trans Fat 0.0g • Cholesterol 80mg • Sodium 190mg • Total Carbohydrate 16g • Dietary Fiber 4g • Sugars 5g • Protein 34 g

Cod Provençal

1 Tbsp	olive oil
1 Tbsp	black pepper
2	plum tomatoes, diced
2	green onions, sliced
4 cloves	garlic, minced
1/4 cup	kalamata olives, chopped
1/4 cup	chopped fresh parsley
2 Tbsp	capers, drained
1/2 tsp	dried red pepper

❖ Preheat oven to 400°F.

❖ In a medium bowl, combine all ingredients.

1 lb	cod fillet

❖ Coat fish with mixture, and arrange in a baking dish. Pour additional mixture over fillets. Bake for 15 minutes or until fish flakes when tested with a fork.

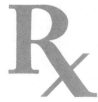

Exchanges/Choices
1 Vegetable • 3 Lean Meat

Calories 150 • Calories from Fat 45 • Total Fat 5.0g • Saturated Fat 0.8g • Trans Fat 0.0g • Cholesterol 50mg • Sodium 270mg • Total Carbohydrate 5g • Dietary Fiber 2g • Sugars 1g • Protein 21 g

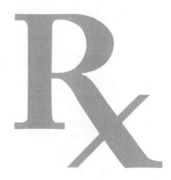

Desserts

Chocolate Rum Cake

Serves 12 / Serving size: 1/12 recipe

2 cups	all-purpose flour
1 tsp	baking soda
1/4 tsp	salt

❖ Preheat oven to 375°F.

❖ In a medium bowl, combine flour, baking soda, and salt.

3 Tbsp	margarine, softened
1/2 cup	packed brown sugar
3/4 cup	unsweetened applesauce
1/2 cup	coffee
3 Tbsp	unsweetened cocoa

❖ In a large bowl, mix margarine, sugar, applesauce, coffee, and cocoa.

1	egg white
1 Tbsp	rum extract
1/2 cup	semi-sweet mini chocolate chips

❖ Add egg white and rum extract; mix until smooth. Add flour mixture, and stir in chocolate chips.

	nonstick cooking spray

❖ Coat an 8-inch square baking pan with cooking spray; spoon batter into pan. Bake for 25 minutes, until a toothpick inserted in the center of the cake comes out clean.

2 Tbsp	powdered sugar

❖ Cool in pan on a wire rack. Remove from pan, and sprinkle with powdered sugar.

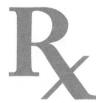

Exchanges/Choices
2 Carbohydrate • 1 Fat

Calories 175 • Calories from Fat 40 • Total Fat 4.5g • Saturated Fat 1.9g • Trans Fat 0.0g • Cholesterol 0mg • Sodium 185mg • Total Carbohydrate 32g • Dietary Fiber 1g • Sugars 15g • Protein 3g

Apple Cake

Serves 12 / Serving size: 1/12 recipe

1 cup	peeled, chopped McIntosh apples
1 cup	peeled, chopped Granny Smith apples
3/4 cup	granulated sugar

❖ Toss apples in sugar; set aside.

❖ Preheat oven to 350°F.

1 cup	all-purpose flour
1/2 cup	whole-wheat flour
1 tsp	baking powder
1/2 tsp	baking soda
1/4 tsp	salt
1 tsp	ground cinnamon
1/2 tsp	allspice

❖ In a large bowl, combine flours, baking powder, baking soda, salt, cinnamon, and allspice.

1/4 cup	canola oil
1	large egg
2 tsp	vanilla

❖ In a separate bowl, combine oil, egg, and vanilla. Add flour mixture to egg mixture. Mix well, and stir in apples.

	nonstick cooking spray

❖ Coat an 8 × 8-inch baking pan with cooking spray. Pour mixture into pan. Bake for 35 minutes, until a toothpick inserted in the center comes out clean. Cool cake in pan on a wire rack.

Exchanges/Choices
2 Carbohydrate • 1 Fat

Calories 160 • Calories from Fat 45 • Total Fat 5.0g • Saturated Fat 0.5g • Trans Fat 0.0g • Cholesterol 20mg • Sodium 140mg • Total Carbohydrate 27g • Dietary Fiber 1g • Sugars 15g • Protein 2g

Peanut Butter Cookies

1 1/4 cups	all-purpose flour
1/2 tsp	salt
1 tsp	baking powder

❖ Preheat oven to 375°F.

❖ In a bowl, mix flour, salt, and baking powder.

1/2 cup	margarine
1/2 cup	smooth peanut butter
1/2 cup	brown sugar
1/2 cup	granulated sugar

❖ In a separate bowl, cream the margarine, peanut butter, and sugars.

1 tsp	vanilla extract
1	large egg

❖ Beat in vanilla and egg. Stir in flour mixture.

❖ Line a cookie sheet with parchment paper. Drop cookies by rounded tablespoons, and flatten each cookie with a fork. Bake 12 minutes, until edges turn slightly brown.

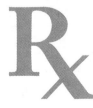

Exchanges/Choices
1 Carbohydrate • 1 Fat

Calories 115 • Calories from Fat 55 • Total Fat 6.0g • Saturated Fat 1.3g • Trans Fat 0.0g • Cholesterol 10mg • Sodium 125mg • Total Carbohydrate 15g • Dietary Fiber 0g • Sugars 9g • Protein 2g

Date Pinwheel Cookies

Serves 24 / Serving size: 2 cookies

1/4 cup	water
1/2 cup	chopped dates
3 Tbsp	granulated sugar

❖ Bring water, dates, and sugar to a boil in a small saucepan. Reduce heat. Cook 2 minutes.

1 Tbsp	lemon juice
1/2 tsp	vanilla

❖ Stir in lemon juice and vanilla. Remove from heat, and set aside.

4 Tbsp	margarine
4 Tbsp	shortening

❖ In a bowl, beat margarine and shortening with an electric mixer for 2 minutes until smooth.

1/4 cup	granulated sugar
1/4 cup	packed brown sugar
1	egg
2 Tbsp	1% milk
1/2 tsp	vanilla

❖ Add sugars, egg, milk, and vanilla.

1 1/2 cups	all-purpose flour
1/4 tsp	baking soda
1/4 tsp	salt

❖ In a separate bowl, combine flour, baking soda, and salt.

❖ Add flour mixture to margarine mixture. Cover and chill for 1 hour.

❖ On a well-floured surface, roll out dough to form a 12 × 10-inch rectangle. Spread date filling over dough. Roll the dough jelly-roll style, brushing off excess flour as you roll. Moisten and pinch edges to seal. Place on a flat surface, and cover with plastic wrap. Refrigerate for at least 2 hours and up to 24 hours.

nonstick cooking spray

❖ Preheat oven to 375°F. Coat a cookie sheet with cooking spray. Cut the dough into 1/4-inch-thick slices. Place slices 2 inches apart on prepared cookie sheet. Bake for 10 minutes, until lightly browned. Remove cookies from cookie sheet, and cool on a wire rack.

Exchanges/Choices
1 Carbohydrate • 1 Fat

Calories 95 • Calories from Fat 30 • Total Fat 3.5g • Saturated Fat 0.9g • Trans Fat 0.0g • Cholesterol 10mg • Sodium 55mg • Total Carbohydrate 14g • Dietary Fiber 0g • Sugars 8g • Protein 1g

Triple Berry Crisp

Serves 6 / Serving size: 1/6 recipe

1/2 cup	*rolled oats*

❖ In a large sauté pan over medium heat, toast oats by stirring 5 minutes until lightly browned. Remove from heat, and transfer oats to a bowl.

1/2 cup	*whole-wheat flour*
1 tsp	*cinnamon*

❖ Add flour and cinnamon to oats; toss well.

1/4 cup	*packed brown sugar*

❖ Add sugar to sauté pan, and cook over low heat, stirring constantly until liquefied.

❖ Slowly blend sugar into oat mixture.

❖ Preheat oven to 400°F.

	nonstick cooking spray

❖ Coat a pie pan with cooking spray.

1 1/2 cups	*strawberries*
3/4 cup	*raspberries*
3/4 cup	*blueberries*
1 tsp	*lemon juice*
1/4 tsp	*vanilla*

❖ Place berries inside pie pan; toss in lemon juice and vanilla. Sprinkle with oat mixture.

❖ Cover pie pan with foil. Bake for 20 minutes. Remove the foil, and bake an additional 5 minutes, until topping is lightly browned.

6 Tbsp	*reduced-fat whipped topping*
6 Tbsp	*fat-free sour cream*

❖ Fold together whipped topping and sour cream.

1 Tbsp	*nutmeg*

❖ Divide berry crisp onto plates, top with whipped topping mixture, and garnish with a sprinkle of nutmeg.

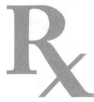

Exchanges/Choices
2 Carbohydrate

Calories 155 • Calories from Fat 20 • Total Fat 2.0g • Saturated Fat 1.0g • Trans Fat 0.0g • Cholesterol 0mg • Sodium 25mg • Total Carbohydrate 33g • Dietary Fiber 5g • Sugars 16g • Protein 4g

Chocolate Chip Granola Bars

nonstick cooking spray

❖ Preheat oven to 400°F.

❖ Coat a 9 × 13-inch pan with cooking spray.

2 cups	rolled oats
1/2 cup	packed brown sugar
1/2 cup	wheat germ
1/4 cup	all-purpose flour
1/4 cup	whole-wheat flour
1/2 tsp	salt
1/2 cup	honey
1	large egg
2 tsp	vanilla
3 oz	chocolate chips

❖ Combine all ingredients, and spread mixture evenly in prepared pan. Bake for 20 minutes.

Exchanges/Choices
2 1/2 Carbohydrate • 1 Fat

Calories 205 • Calories from Fat 35 • Total Fat 4.0g • Saturated Fat 1.6g • Trans Fat 0.0g • Cholesterol 20mg • Sodium 110mg • Total Carbohydrate 40g • Dietary Fiber 3g • Sugars 25g • Protein 5g

Peach Tart

	nonstick cooking spray

❖ Preheat oven to 375°F.

❖ Coat a pie pan with cooking spray.

1	29-oz can sliced peaches in water, drained

❖ Place peaches in pie pan.

1 cup	rolled oats, lightly toasted
1/2 cup	nonfat milk
2	large eggs
3 Tbsp	molasses
2 tsp	vanilla
1/2 tsp	nutmeg

❖ In a bowl, combine oats, milk, eggs, molasses, vanilla, and nutmeg. Mix well. Pour over peaches.

❖ Bake for 30 minutes, until golden brown.

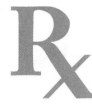

Exchanges/Choices
2 Carbohydrate • 1/2 Fat

Calories 150 • Calories from Fat 20 • Total Fat 2.5g • Saturated Fat 0.7g • Trans Fat 0.0g • Cholesterol 70mg • Sodium 40mg • Total Carbohydrate 26g • Dietary Fiber 3g • Sugars 14g • Protein 5g

Blueberry Pie

	nonstick cooking spray

❖ Preheat oven to 350°F.

❖ Coat a pie pan with cooking spray.

6	*9 × 14-inch sheets phyllo dough*
	nonstick cooking spray

❖ Line the pie pan with phyllo sheets, lightly coating each one with cooking spray to prevent them from drying out. Bake pie shell for 15 minutes, until lightly browned. Remove from oven, and let cool on wire rack.

20 oz	*fresh blueberries*
1 Tbsp	*sugar*
2 tsp	*margarine*
1 1/2 tsp	*lemon juice*

❖ In a saucepan over medium heat, combine blueberries, sugar, and margarine. Cook, stirring frequently, until sugar has dissolved. Stir in lemon juice. Remove from heat, and let cool. Place blueberry mixture into prepared pie shell.

8 oz	*low-fat blueberry yogurt*
1/2 cup	*light frozen whipped topping, thawed*

❖ Spread yogurt on top of pie, and top with whipped cream.

Exchanges/Choices
1 1/2 Carbohydrate • 1/2 Fat

Calories 120 • Calories from Fat 20 • Total Fat 2.0g • Saturated Fat 0.8g • Trans Fat 0.0g • Cholesterol 0mg • Sodium 60mg • Total Carbohydrate 24g • Dietary Fiber 2g • Sugars 15g • Protein 2g

Lemon Poppy Cake

	nonstick cooking spray

❖ Preheat oven to 350°F.

❖ Coat an 8 × 6-inch pan with cooking spray.

6 Tbsp	margarine
1 cup	granulated sugar

❖ In a large bowl, cream the margarine and sugar.

2	large eggs

❖ Add eggs one at a time, mixing well after each addition.

2 Tbsp	lemon juice
1/4 cup	low-fat plain yogurt
1 Tbsp	grated lemon peel
1/4 cup	poppy seeds

❖ Stir in lemon juice, yogurt, lemon peel, and poppy seeds.

3/4 cup	all-purpose flour
3/4 cup	whole-wheat flour
3/4 tsp	baking soda
1/4 tsp	salt

❖ Add flours, baking soda, and salt; mix until well blended.

❖ Pour into prepared pan, and bake for 50 minutes, until a toothpick inserted in the center comes out clean. Cool on a wire rack.

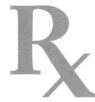

Exchanges/Choices
2 Carbohydrate • 1 Fat

Calories 185 • Calories from Fat 55 • Total Fat 6.0g • Saturated Fat 1.5g • Trans Fat 0.0g • Cholesterol 35mg • Sodium 190mg • Total Carbohydrate 30g • Dietary Fiber 2g • Sugars 17g • Protein 4g

Spicy Popcorn

Serves 4 / Serving size: 1/4 recipe

2 Tbsp	margarine, melted
4 cups	air-popped popcorn

❖ Drizzle margarine over popcorn, and toss well to coat.

1/2 tsp	salt
1/4 tsp	chili powder
1/4 tsp	garlic powder
1/4 tsp	onion powder

❖ Combine salt and chili, garlic, and onion powders. Sprinkle over popcorn. Toss again to coat.

Exchanges/Choices
1/2 Starch • 1 Fat

Calories 70 • Calories from Fat 40 • Total Fat 4.5g • Saturated Fat 1.1g • Trans Fat 0.0g • Cholesterol 0mg • Sodium 340mg • Total Carbohydrate 7g • Dietary Fiber 1g • Sugars 0g • Protein 1g

Simply Smoothie

Serves 4 / Serving size: 1/4 recipe

3/4 cup	orange juice
2	bananas
1 cup	sliced strawberries
1 cup	nonfat vanilla yogurt
1/2 cup	ice

❖ Combine all ingredients in a blender. Cover and blend until smooth.

Exchanges/Choices
2 Fruit

Calories 115 • Calories from Fat 5 • Total Fat 0.5g • Saturated Fat 0.2g • Trans Fat 0.0g • Cholesterol 0mg • Sodium 30mg • Total Carbohydrate 28g • Dietary Fiber 3g • Sugars 17g • Protein 3g

Simply Chocolate Smoothie

Serves 4 / Serving size: 1/4 recipe

1/2 cup	nonfat milk
2	bananas
3 Tbsp	unsweetened cocoa powder
1 cup	nonfat vanilla yogurt
1/2 cup	ice

❖ Combine all ingredients in a blender. Cover and blend until smooth.

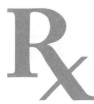

Exchanges/Choices
1 Fruit • 1/2 Fat-Free Milk

Calories 100 • Calories from Fat 10 • Total Fat 1.0g • Saturated Fat 0.5g • Trans Fat 0.0g • Cholesterol 0mg • Sodium 40mg • Total Carbohydrate 24g • Dietary Fiber 3g • Sugars 13g • Protein 4g

Melon Granita

Serves 6 / Serving size: 1/6 recipe

3 cups	cubed honeydew
3 cups	cubed watermelon
3 cups	cubed cantaloupe

❖ Remove seeds from melons, and cut each melon into large cubes.

3 Tbsp	granulated sugar
3 Tbsp	lemon juice

❖ Place cubes of one type of melon in a blender or food processor, and purée. Stir in 1 Tbsp sugar and 1 Tbsp lemon juice for each melon type. Repeat for each melon type. Pour melon mixtures into individual nonreactive metal baking pans.

❖ Freeze for 3 hours before serving.

Exchanges/Choices
2 Fruit

Calories 105 • Calories from Fat 0 • Total Fat 0.0g • Saturated Fat 0.1g • Trans Fat 0.0g • Cholesterol 0mg • Sodium 30mg • Total Carbohydrate 27g • Dietary Fiber 2g • Sugars 24g • Protein 2g

Carrot Cake

Serves 16 / Serving size: 1/16 recipe

	nonstick cooking spray

❖ Coat a fluted tube pan with cooking spray; set aside.

❖ Preheat oven to 350°F.

1/2 cup	margarine, softened
1 cup	granulated sugar
3/4 cup	packed brown sugar

❖ In a large bowl, cream the margarine and sugars.

2	large eggs

❖ Add eggs one at a time, mixing well after each addition.

1/4 cup	applesauce
1 Tbsp	vanilla
3 cups	shredded carrots
1 1/2 cups	all-purpose flour
1 cup	whole-wheat flour
1 tsp	baking powder
1/2 tsp	cinnamon

❖ Add applesauce, vanilla, carrots, flours, baking powder, and cinnamon. Mix until well blended.

1/2 cup	chopped black walnuts

❖ Stir in walnuts.

❖ Pour batter into prepared pan, and bake for 1 hour. Cool cake on wire rack.

4 oz	fat-free cream cheese
1 Tbsp	fat-free sour cream
5 tsp	powdered sugar

❖ Combine cream cheese, sour cream, and powdered sugar; mix well. Stir until smooth. Spread mixture over cooled cake.

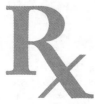

Exchanges/Choices
3 Carbohydrate • 1 1/2 Fat

Calories 270 • Calories from Fat 90 • Total Fat 10.0g • Saturated Fat 1.6g • Trans Fat 0.0g • Cholesterol 30mg • Sodium 140mg • Total Carbohydrate 42g • Dietary Fiber 2g • Sugars 25g • Protein 6g

Chocolate Almond Biscotti

	nonstick cooking spray

❖ Preheat oven to 350°F. Coat a large baking pan with cooking spray.

3	*large eggs*
1 tsp	*grated orange peel*
1 tsp	*vanilla extract*

❖ In a large bowl, combine eggs, orange peel, and vanilla extract.

1 1/2 cups	*all-purpose flour*
1/2 cup	*whole-wheat flour*
1 cup	*granulated sugar*
1/2 cup	*unsweetened cocoa powder*
1 tsp	*baking soda*
1/2 tsp	*salt*

❖ In a separate bowl, combine flours, sugar, cocoa powder, baking soda, and salt.

1/4 cup	*semi-sweet chocolate chips*
1/2 cup	*almonds, toasted*

❖ Add flour mixture to egg mixture. Stir in chocolate chips and almonds. Divide the dough in half.

❖ On a well-floured surface, roll dough halves into a 14-inch length by 2-inch width. Bake for 50 minutes, until golden brown. Remove from oven, and let cool for 5 minutes. Lower the oven temperature to 275°F. Using a serrated knife, cut strips diagonally into 1/2-inch slices. Place the slices cut side down on baking sheet, turning over halfway through the baking time, until golden brown and crisp, 25 minutes. Cool biscotti on a wire rack.

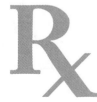

Exchanges/Choices
1 Carbohydrate • 1/2 Fat

Calories 105 • Calories from Fat 25 • Total Fat 3.0g • Saturated Fat 0.8g • Trans Fat 0.0g • Cholesterol 25mg • Sodium 105mg • Total Carbohydrate 18g • Dietary Fiber 2g • Sugars 9g • Protein 3g

Stuffed Baked Peaches

Serves 8 / Serving size: 1/8 recipe

4	*medium peaches*

❖ Preheat oven to 400°F.

❖ Halve peaches, and remove pits. Cut a thin slice from each bottom half to prevent them from rolling over. Scoop out one tablespoon of flesh from each half, chop coarsely, and set aside. Place the peach halves in a baking dish large enough to just fit the eight halves.

1 cup	*cranberries, chopped*
1/3 cup	*packed brown sugar*
2 Tbsp	*all-purpose flour*
1 tsp	*vanilla extract*
1/2 cup	*rolled oats*

❖ In a bowl, combine chopped peaches, cranberries, sugar, flour, vanilla extract, and oats. Divide mixture into each peach half.

2 Tbsp	*margarine*
1/4 cup	*water*

❖ Cut margarine into eight pieces, and place one piece on top of each half. Pour water into the bottom of the pan. Bake for 25 minutes.

4 Tbsp	*fat-free sour cream*

❖ Pour any juices over baked peach halves, and top with sour cream.

Exchanges/Choices
1 1/2 Carbohydrate • 1/2 Fat

Calories 120 • Calories from Fat 20 • Total Fat 2.5g • Saturated Fat 0.6g • Trans Fat 0.0g • Cholesterol 0mg • Sodium 35mg • Total Carbohydrate 24g • Dietary Fiber 2g • Sugars 16g • Protein 2g

Apricot Crème Brûlée

2 cups	evaporated nonfat milk
1/4 cup	granulated sugar
1 tsp	vanilla extract
1 Tbsp	arrowroot

❖ Preheat oven to 350°F.

❖ In a saucepan, add milk, sugar, vanilla, and arrowroot. Slowly bring to a boil until thickened, stirring occasionally. Remove from heat.

4	egg whites
1	large egg
1/4 cup	granulated sugar

❖ In a bowl, whisk egg whites, egg, and sugar. Slowly add evaporated milk mixture to the egg mixture.

1	15-oz can apricots in water, drained

❖ Divide apricots among six 6-oz ramekins. Portion the mixture on top of apricots. Place ramekins in a shallow large pan. Fill the pan with water to 3/4 of the height of the ramekins. Bake for 1 hour, until custard is set in the center. Carefully remove from oven, and let cool.

❖ Tightly wrap custard, and refrigerate overnight.

2 Tbsp	granulated sugar

❖ To serve, sprinkle each serving with 1 tsp sugar, and place under broiler until golden brown.

Exchanges/Choices
1/2 Fat-Free Milk • 2 Carbohydrate

Calories 195 • Calories from Fat 10 • Total Fat 1.0g • Saturated Fat 0.4g • Trans Fat 0.0g • Cholesterol 40mg • Sodium 150mg • Total Carbohydrate 37g • Dietary Fiber 1g • Sugars 34g • Protein 10g

Bread Pudding

	nonstick cooking spray

❖ Preheat oven to 350°F.

❖ Coat an 8-inch round cake pan with cooking spray.

3/4 lb	stale whole-wheat bread

❖ Cut the bread into 1-inch cubes. Lightly toast the bread in the oven for 5 minutes. Reduce heat to 325°F.

1/2 cup	raisins

❖ Combine toasted bread with raisins, and place in prepared pan.

1 1/2 cups	nonfat milk
3	eggs, beaten
1/3 cup	granulated sugar

❖ In a bowl, combine milk, eggs, and sugar. Mix well, and pour over bread. Place cake pan in a shallow large pan. Fill larger pan with water to 3/4 of the height of the cake pan. Bake for 45 minutes until custard is set. The custard will be firm but will still jiggle when gently shaken. Remove from oven, and let cool in the water bath.

Exchanges/Choices
2 1/2 Carbohydrate • 1/2 Fat

Calories 205 • Calories from Fat 30 • Total Fat 3.5g • Saturated Fat 0.9g • Trans Fat 0.3g • Cholesterol 80mg • Sodium 245mg • Total Carbohydrate 35g • Dietary Fiber 3g • Sugars 18g • Protein 10g

Pastry Cream with Kiwi Topping

2	egg yolks
1	large egg
3 Tbsp	cornstarch

❖ In a bowl, beat egg yolks and whole egg. Sift cornstarch into the eggs. Beat until smooth.

| 1/2 cup | granulated sugar |
| 2 cups | nonfat milk |

❖ In a saucepan, combine sugar and milk, and bring just to a boil. In a thin stream, slowly beat hot milk into egg mixture. Return mixture to the heat, and bring to a boil, stirring constantly until thickened. Remove from heat.

| 2 Tbsp | margarine |
| 1 1/2 tsp | vanilla extract |

❖ Stir in margarine and vanilla until margarine is melted and completely blended in.

❖ Divide cream among eight individual serving dishes. Tightly cover with plastic wrap to prevent a crust from forming. Refrigerate for 2 hours until cooled.

| 4 | fresh kiwi, peeled and sliced |

❖ Place sliced kiwi over cream in individual dishes.

| 3 Tbsp | apricot preserves |

❖ In a small saucepan, warm apricot preserves. Brush the glaze on the kiwi to coat completely.

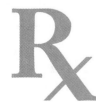

Exchanges/Choices
2 Carbohydrate • 1 Fat

Calories 165 • Calories from Fat 35 • Total Fat 4.0g • Saturated Fat 1.1g • Trans Fat 0.0g • Cholesterol 80mg • Sodium 65mg • Total Carbohydrate 29g • Dietary Fiber 1g • Sugars 23g • Protein 4g

Oatmeal Cookies

1/2 cup	margarine
1/2 cup	packed brown sugar
1/4 cup	granulated sugar
1	large egg
1 tsp	vanilla

❖ Preheat oven to 350°F.

❖ Beat together margarine and sugars until creamy. Add egg and vanilla.

1/2 cup	all-purpose flour
1/4 cup	whole-wheat flour
1/2 tsp	baking soda
1/4 tsp	cinnamon

❖ Beat in flours, baking soda, and cinnamon.

2 1/2 cups	rolled oats
1/2 cup	golden raisins

❖ Stir in oats and raisins. Mix well. Drop by rounded teaspoonfuls onto an ungreased cookie sheet.

1/4 cup	granulated sugar

❖ Dip the bottom of a round glass into the sugar, and press down on each cookie to flatten slightly. Bake for 10 minutes, until golden brown. Cook on a wire rack.

Exchanges/Choices
2 Carbohydrate • 1/2 Fat

Calories 155 • Calories from Fat 40 • Total Fat 4.5g • Saturated Fat 1.1g • Trans Fat 0.0g • Cholesterol 10mg • Sodium 85mg • Total Carbohydrate 26g • Dietary Fiber 2g • Sugars 14g • Protein 3g

Brownies

4 Tbsp	*margarine*

❖ Preheat oven to 350°F.

❖ In a small saucepan, melt margarine and remove from heat.

1/2 cup	*granulated sugar*
1 Tbsp	*vanilla extract*

❖ Stir in sugar and vanilla extract.

1 cup	*all-purpose flour*
4 Tbsp	*unsweetened cocoa powder*
1 tsp	*baking powder*

❖ Stir in flour, cocoa, and baking powder. Do not overmix.

1/3 cup	*semi-sweet mini chocolate chips*

❖ Stir in chocolate chips.

	nonstick cooking spray

❖ Spray an 8 × 8-inch baking pan with cooking spray, and pour batter evenly into pan. Bake for 20 minutes, until a toothpick inserted in the center comes out clean. Cool on a wire rack.

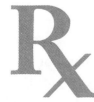

Exchanges/Choices
1 Carbohydrate • 1/2 Fat

Calories 95 • Calories from Fat 30 • Total Fat 3.5g • Saturated Fat 1.3g • Trans Fat 0.0g • Cholesterol 0mg • Sodium 45mg • Total Carbohydrate 15g • Dietary Fiber 1g • Sugars 8g • Protein 1g

Marble Pound Cake

nonstick cooking spray

❖ Preheat oven to 350°F.

❖ Coat an 8 × 6-inch loaf pan with cooking spray.

6 Tbsp	*margarine*
1 cup	*granulated sugar*
1 tsp	*vanilla extract*
1 Tbsp	*water*

❖ In a bowl, mix margarine and sugar until creamy. Add vanilla extract and water.

2	*large eggs*
1 1/2 cup	*sifted all-purpose flour*
1/4 tsp	*baking soda*

❖ Add eggs one at a time, mixing well after each addition. Add flour and baking soda. Mix until just blended in.

2 Tbsp	*unsweetened cocoa powder*

❖ Place half of the batter in a separate bowl, and add cocoa. Mix well.

❖ Fill loaf pan with alternating layers of plain and chocolate batters. Run a knife through the batter to marble the mixture. Bake for 55 minutes, until a toothpick inserted in the center comes out clean. Cool on a wire rack.

Exchanges/Choices
2 Carbohydrate • 1 Fat

Calories 170 • Calories from Fat 45 • Total Fat 5.0g • Saturated Fat 1.4g • Trans Fat 0.0g • Cholesterol 35mg • Sodium 65mg • Total Carbohydrate 29g • Dietary Fiber 1g • Sugars 17g • Protein 3g

Angel Food Cake

Serves 12 / Serving size: 1/12 recipe

| 1/3 cup | sifted all-purpose flour |
| 1 cup | granulated sugar |

❖ Preheat oven to 350°F.

❖ Sift flour with sugar; set aside.

5	egg whites, at room temperature
1/4 tsp	salt
1/2 tsp	cream of tartar

❖ Beat egg whites, salt, and cream of tartar until they form soft peaks.

1 cup	granulated sugar
1/2 tsp	vanilla extract
1/4 tsp	almond extract

❖ Gradually beat in sugar and extracts. Fold flour mixture into egg mixture until it is thoroughly absorbed.

❖ Fill an 8-inch ungreased angel food pan with batter. Bake for 30 minutes. Cool upside down on cooling rack for at least an hour before removing from pan.

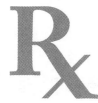

Exchanges/Choices
2 1/2 Carbohydrate

Calories 150 • Calories from Fat 0 • Total Fat 0.0g • Saturated Fat 0.0g • Trans Fat 0.0g • Cholesterol 0mg • Sodium 70mg • Total Carbohydrate 36g • Dietary Fiber 0g • Sugars 34g • Protein 2g

Jelly Rolls

4	eggs, separated and whites reserved
2	egg yolks
3 Tbsp	grated orange peel
1/4 cup	granulated sugar

❖ Preheat oven to 425°F.

❖ Line a 15 × 10-inch cake pan with parchment paper.

❖ Combine 6 egg yolks, orange peel, and sugar. Beat 5 minutes until creamy.

1/4 cup	granulated sugar

❖ In a separate bowl, beat 4 egg whites and sugar until stiff. Fold egg-white mixture into egg-yolk mixture.

3/4 cup	all-purpose flour
1/2 tsp	baking powder

❖ Sift flour with baking powder, and fold into egg mixture. Spread batter evenly into the prepared pan. Bake for 10 minutes, until a toothpick inserted in center comes out clean.

1/2 cup	powdered sugar

❖ Spread a kitchen towel on a clean surface, and sprinkle it with powdered sugar. Turn the cake upside down onto the towel, and remove the parchment paper. Roll the cake up with the towel inside of it. Let the rolled cake cool on a wire rack.

3/4 cup	100% fruit, seedless raspberry jam

❖ Unroll the cake, and spread jam over the surface.

1/4 cup	powdered sugar

❖ Reroll the cake without the towel, and sift powdered sugar on top. Cut the cake into 10 1-inch slices.

Exchanges/Choices
2 1/2 Carbohydrate • 1/2 Fat

Calories 195 • Calories from Fat 25 • Total Fat 3.0g • Saturated Fat 1.0g • Trans Fat 0.0g • Cholesterol 125mg • Sodium 55mg • Total Carbohydrate 39g • Dietary Fiber 1g • Sugars 29g • Protein 4g

Meringue Cookies

2	*egg whites*
1/2 tsp	*vanilla*
1/4 tsp	*cream of tartar*

❖ Preheat oven to 300°F.

❖ Line a large baking pan with parchment paper. Draw 3-inch circles 1 inch apart from each other onto the parchment paper.

❖ In a bowl, beat egg whites, vanilla, and cream of tartar until soft peaks form.

1/2 cup	*granulated sugar*

❖ Gradually add sugar, and beat until stiff peaks form.

❖ Put egg-white mixture in a decorating bag fitted with a 1/4-inch round tip. Fill bag half full. Beginning at the center of the circle, squeeze the bag gently in a spiral until the circle is filled. Release pressure as you pull up the tip.

1 cup	*slivered almonds*

❖ Top each cookie with almonds. Bake for 15 minutes. Turn off the oven, and let the cookies rest with the door closed for 30 minutes.

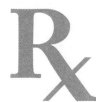

Exchanges/Choices
1/2 Carbohydrate • 1 Fat

Calories 90 • Calories from Fat 45 • Total Fat 5.0g • Saturated Fat 0.4g • Trans Fat 0.0g • Cholesterol 0mg • Sodium 10mg • Total Carbohydrate 10g • Dietary Fiber 1g • Sugars 9g • Protein 3g

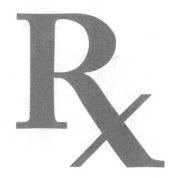

Index

ALPHABETICAL LIST OF RECIPES

RECIPES BY SUBJECT

Other Titles from the American Diabetes Association

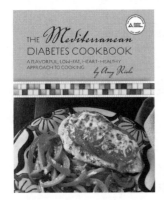

The Mediterranean Diabetes Cookbook
by Amy Riolo

Mediterranean cuisine uses healthful, fresh ingredients, and when it is paired with the moderate Mediterranean lifestyle, you can enjoy delicious, traditional, and naturally diabetes-friendly dishes. Award-winning food writer Amy Riolo introduces you to a new world of health, well-being, and flavor. Leave behind tired, watered-down diabetes recipes and regain the joys of eating.
Order no. 4674-01; $19.95

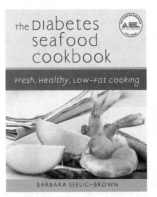

The Diabetes Seafood Cookbook
by Barbara Seelig-Brown

Seafood is the perfect choice for anyone looking to eat healthfully without skimping on flavor. From freshwater and saltwater fish to crab, shrimp, and clams, this book delivers over 150 delicious recipes for the perfect party appetizer, a delightful family dinner, or a satisfying side dish.
Order no. 4670.01; Price $18.95

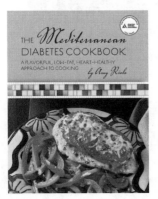

Diabetes Meal Planning Made Easy, 4th Edition
by Hope S. Warshaw, MMSc, RD, CDE, BC-ADM

This new edition of the meal-planning bestseller uncovers the secrets to healthy eating with diabetes— from the basics of what to eat to the practical skills of shopping, planning nutritious meals, and even eating healthy restaurant meals. You don't have to change your life to eat healthy, but you might be surprised to learn how eating healthy can change your life!
Order no. 4706-04; Price $16.95

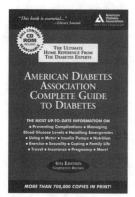
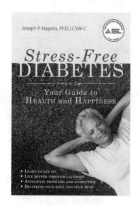
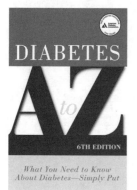